BODY INTELLIGENCE

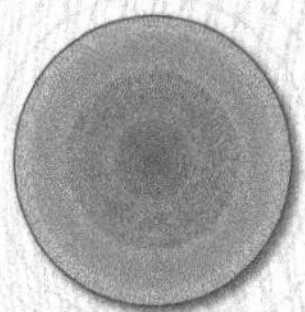 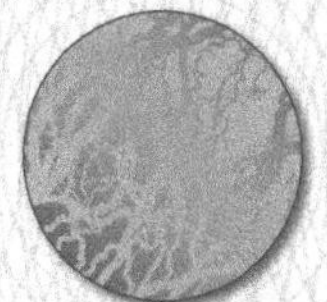 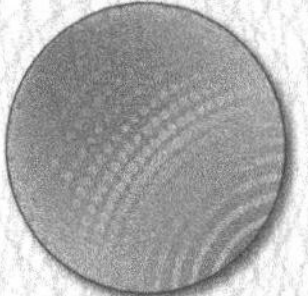 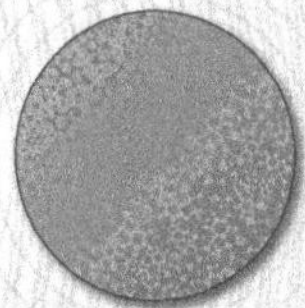

BODY INTELLIGENCE

Harness Your Body's Energies for Your Best Life

JOSEPH CARDILLO, PhD

ATRIA PAPERBACK
New York London Toronto Sydney New Delhi

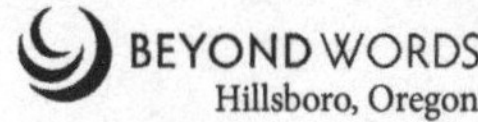

Hillsboro, Oregon

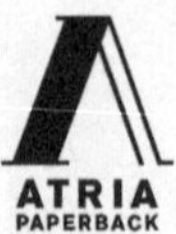

ATRIA PAPERBACK
An Imprint of Simon & Schuster, Inc.
1230 Avenue of the Americas
New York, NY 10020

BEYOND WORDS
20827 N.W. Cornell Road, Suite 500
Hillsboro, Oregon 97124-9808
503-531-8700 / 503-531-8773 fax
www.beyondword.com

Managing editor: Lindsay S. Easterbrooks-Brown
Editor: Anna Noak, Sarah Heilman
Copyeditor: Michelle Blair
Proofreader: Jennifer Weaver-Neist
Design: Devon Smith
Composition: William H. Brunson Typography Services

First Atria Books/Beyond Words paperback edition September 2017

Manufactured in the United States of America

10 9 8 7 6 5 4 3 2 1

The Library of Congress has cataloged the hardcover edition as follows:

Cardillo, Joseph,
Body intelligence : harness your body's energies for your best life / Joseph Cardillo.
pages cm
1. Self-actualization (Psychology). 2. Mind and body. I. Title.
BF637.S4C3557 2015
158.1—dc23

2015015373

ISBN: 978-1-58270-518-7 (hc)
ISBN: 978-1-58270-519-4 (pbk)
ISBN: 978-1-4767-8225-6 (eBook)

The corporate mission of Beyond Words Publishing, Inc.: *Inspire to Integrity*

For my wife, Elaine,
and our daughters, Isabella and Veronica,
whom we loved before they were born,

and to my father and mother,
Alfio and Josephine Cardillo

The secret of change is to focus all of your energy,
not on fighting the old but on building the new.

—Dan Millman

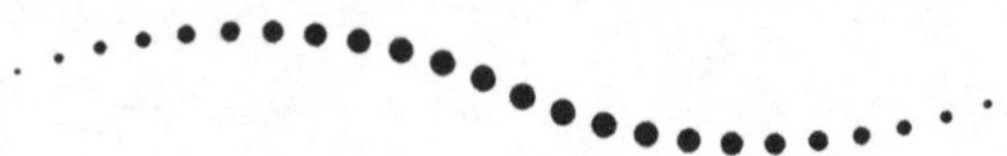

DISCLAIMER

The case examples in this book are drawn from media accounts or are composite examples based upon behaviors encountered in the author's own professional experiences. None of the individuals described were clients. The names and details have been changed to protect the privacy of the people involved. This publication does not claim medical advice. It is not intended as a substitute for the advice of healthcare professionals.

Before engaging in any physical, psychological, or spiritual training programs, you should always check with your physicians and other professional healthcare providers to be sure that they are right for you.

CONTENTS

INTRODUCTION

I wish that all of nature's magnificence, the emotion of the land, the living energy of place could be photographed.

—Annie Leibovitz

You are energy, your world is energy, and everything in your world is energy. What allows you to experience others and for them to experience you is energy. What followed you into this life is energy, and what will usher you out is energy.

One thing we all want is more and better quality *energy*. You get caught in the whirlwind of daily activities and, at the end of the day, go to bed drained or with your mind racing, or both. We wonder where we are ever going to get the energy for all those things we really want to do.

Part of the problem is that we have been conditioned to think there are only two kinds of energy: high and low. As a result, many individuals turn to energy drinks, supplements, and other substances to bring them either "up" or "down"—all of which can have harmful side effects and often leave you with less overall energy than before.

Your energy, however, like your sleep rhythms, is cyclical, and you need your natural energy dips in order to soar. But you also want to be able to regulate those dips so that when you need to be "on," you can get yourself there naturally and fast.

In order to do this, you need to understand that energy is more complex than simply being high or low. Instead, *energy* is the combination of information and force—also known as *informed power*. Information can direct force in any number of ways, meaning that there are also many different and specific types of energy—far more than those that make you feel excited or mellow.

The ways you understand and process a particular energy will factor into how effective it is for you as well. Your mind and body operate optimally when you match specific daily tasks with the best type of energy for the job. The specific energy you need may be calming, arousing, pain relieving, memory enhancing, creative, or any of the numerous kinds of energy out there.

For example, a weightlifter about to bench-press 350 pounds uses a different sort of energy than a business manager who has to complete a PowerPoint presentation for the next day. Ditto for the math student poring over a difficult equation, or the romantic partner struggling to heal a broken heart. Matching your goal with the right energy will, in large part, determine the success, ease, and personal satisfaction you derive from any activity and from life in general.

Think about your favorite hobby or activity. Now imagine yourself engaging in that activity and loving whatever you are doing so thoroughly you lose track of time, limitations, and stressors. This effect is what occurs when you match the right energy with the right task. It is a hallmark of balanced energy. When your mind and body are synced this way, you're not even thinking "life doesn't get any better than this." You naturally feel that way all over. You are living it.

At its best, your mental and physical energy will enable you to live this vivid and brilliantly experienced life.

When you live this way, you flow through all you do, and you experience more in every way—physically, cognitively, emotionally, spiritually, and socially. You feel your influence on other people and environments and theirs on you. Your life purpose and the power you need to achieve it become clearer and available to you. You become vividly present, focused, and accurate in your thoughts, feelings, and actions. You not only feel but are stronger, healthier, and happier. You flow. Ultimately, your own personal energy evolves and keeps evolving.

The Intention of This Book

Body Intelligence and all of the information in it is intended to help you achieve that vivid, brilliantly experienced life. A major part of achieving this life is learning to identify and utilize the energy resources available to you. This skill will be a main focus throughout this book; and as we explore using energy to reach the full potential of your whole living being, we will discuss the mechanisms within your body and mind that enable you to consciously connect and interact with the energies that surround and permeate your life (as well as the lives of others). You will learn how these mechanisms enable you to regulate these energies to enhance your daily activities with the specific force and information you need, when you need it.

You will also learn how to keep negative energies at bay, preventing many health concerns (physical, mental, social, and spiritual) from gaining root in your life or affecting your daily events.

Additionally, you will learn how to train your mind to hit that sweet spot of high-quality energy and sustain it so that it aids you in all your daily endeavors.

With a little practice, you'll start sailing through your day; sleeping better at night; and waking up feeling refreshed, healthy, and ready to go. You will feel more like yourself and enjoy yourself (as well as others) more. As you code this synchronization into your mind and body by making it a daily practice, you will notice that you flow into deeper and longer-lasting satisfaction, personal and interpersonal development, and peace. This is the ultimate goal of this book: to enable you to use your energy and the energy around you to heighten your spirit, and bring more peace and love into your life and into all realms of life that surround you. May the concepts and tools described within these pages serve you well.

1

WHAT IS ENERGY?

Once we begin to change our perception, our thinking,
it's amazing how other things in our lives start changing also.
The domino effect begins with the first step within ourselves.
It's not esoteric; it's human energy.

—Kingsley Dennis

Just what is this thing we call *energy* and how does it affect our performance? What can we do with energy to live fuller, happier, healthier lives?

Scientists have been telling us for over a century that all things are made of energy. All of life, from bacteria to trees to the Universe at large, holds and requires energy to exist. In the very first cells that made you *you* and in all you will do, energy is there—utilized and required.

Even what appears as solid mass is nothing but a form of energy. Even an object at rest has energy stored within. The relationship between the two (energy and solid mass) is conveyed in Einstein's famous equation, $e=mc^2$, which fundamentally changed the way we see and experience our world. His equation provided a recipe, so to speak, for how much energy is necessary to create the "appearance" of mass. As Lynne McTaggart writes in her book *The Field*, "It means that there aren't two fundamental physical entities—something material and another immaterial—but only one: energy."[1]

This corresponds with the idea that even empty space, which makes up 96 percent of our Universe, is seething with energy. In another work of McTaggart's, she cites Nobel laureate-physicist Dr. Richard Feynman, who remarked that "the energy in a cubic meter of space was enough to boil all the oceans of the world."[2]

From the perspective of holistic medicine, what this all comes down to is that everything you touch, hear, taste, see, smell, think, say, or feel—essentially, anything you experience at all—is, at its most fundamental level, energy interacting with other energy.

This precious current, which preceded our birth and ushered us into this life, flows with us through all we do in it and keeps on flowing even after we pass. Learning to regulate it will make positive and significant changes in your life because it gives you a tangible way to shape the quality of all you do (as well as help others do the same) by using life's most plentiful and basic resource. But what exactly can we do with this energy?

Your Body's Energetic Tour de Force

Energy empowers the body to get things done—everything from having a thought to walking across the room, eating a meal, or writing a piece of music. The energy used by your body comes in various forms, including light, chemical, electric, heat, sound, and mechanical energy. You can use each type to balance or intensify the others, and sometimes, you can even substitute one for another that might be lacking.

Light energy, for example, transferred from the sun and into our environment, is transformed into *chemical energy* within the foods that we eat and within the body itself. *Electrical energy*, generally speaking, is generated at the cellular level via chemical (sodium, potassium) interactions within the body. It is another primary source of power for the body—like when your nervous system streams messages, via electrical impulses, which help you regulate a wide range of functions, such as balancing *intracellular environments* (inside the cell) and *intercellular communication* (between cells). It is also crucial to the firing of neurotransmitters, which help regulate your heart rate, muscle movement, and moods, and can even guide your thoughts. We use *heat*, or *thermal energy* (which is transformed from chemical energy and also derived as a byproduct of *mechanical energy*), for maintaining body temperature, and helping our body release toxins and alleviate mental and physical stress. Mechanical energy is energy that empowers your movement. With regard to the body, it can be understood as *potential energy* because of its positioning (like a baseball pitcher's cocked arm or an archer's drawn-back bow) or *kinetic energy* because it is in motion (like the pitcher's moving arm or the flying baseball). *Sound energy* is produced when something vibrates and makes sound waves (like the sound of breath passing through our lips or blood streaming through an umbilical cord).

These forms of energy generate an integrated power base that does everything from helping us physically move around to coordinating the flow of information through every part of our bodies.

Energy = Force and Information

In mind-body medicine, when we use the term *energy*, we are referring to the combination of information and force—what we can define as *informed power*. (Information refers to patterns, form, structure, and other data.) Information gives design or purpose to force. Force can be understood as the capacity to do work or overcome resistance. From the smallest to the biggest thing you can imagine, whether it is a subatomic particle or an entire universe, everything requires force to exist, as well as to do anything.

As a simple example, when you feel like something in your environment or life is motivating you (force) in a specific way (information) to get up on your feet, to be alert, or to do anything, energetically speaking, it probably is. Perhaps you receive a letter from your grandmother and you then feel the motivation to bake cupcakes. This phenomenon can take unlimited forms and that "something" can be any energy source, from you (or someone else) tapping out a beat with your fingers to bumping into an old friend you haven't seen in a while.

Each of these energy events involves both force and information to which your mind and body react. As a result, they can change your life, both for the short and long term. You can learn to control this dynamic using energetic changes to guide you in a positive direction, in sync with your needs and goals, or you can choose to ignore it. The choice is yours. Either way, you are subject to it, and as a result, you are ever changing: biologically, mentally, and spiritually.

Same Thing, Different Package

Historically, many world traditions have emphasized the cultivation of energy from various sources—physical, psychic (mental/emotional), and spiritual—for purposes of health and better, longer, more positive living. This concept, for instance, has been a core idea in Asian medicines and philosophies for millennia.

Interestingly, thousands of years later, Western medicine is delivering a similar message: the energy, or informed power, you cultivate and stream through your body and mind determines who and what you are, as well as how healthfully, satisfyingly, and successfully you live. Furthermore, how you do this determines what input you have in what you become. If you do not cultivate informed power, it will still make all of these determinations, yet you will have abdicated your freedom to manage them. Body intelligence is your awareness of the energetic messages your body is sending you about the performance of your body and mind and how you listen and respond to them.

From the perspective of mind-body medicine (as well as that of other alternative medicines), the body and mind, like the Universe, are fundamentally alike—that is, they are made of pure energy, force, and information. Deepak Chopra, in his book *Ageless Body, Timeless Mind*, states that:

> Your body appears to be composed of solid matter that can be broken down into molecules and atoms, but quantum physics tells us that every atom is more than 99.9999 percent empty space, and subatomic particles moving at lightning speed through this space are actually bundles of vibrating energy. These vibrations aren't random and meaningless, however; they carry information.[3]

What is key in all of these concepts is that through the mind-body connection, you can begin to regulate the physical, mental, and spiritual energy that is influencing you at any given moment in order to achieve a wide range of specific daily effects.

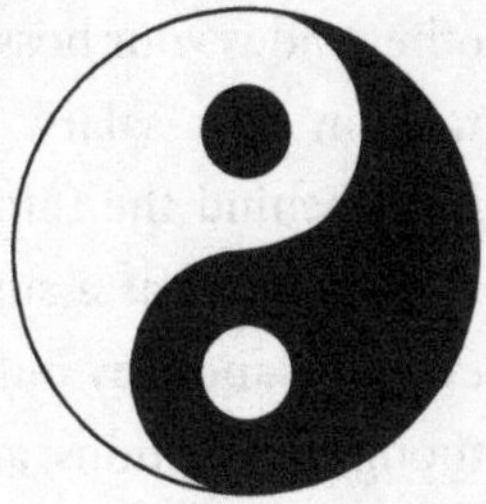

A core principle of mind-body medicine (and traditional Chinese medicine) is the idea of *yin* and *yang*, which serves as an example of taking medicine to the quantum zone. In the *yin-yang principle*, yin provides the information patterns while yang represents the force, both of which are needed for us to grow physically, mentally, and spiritually. Much like Chopra's explanation of energy containing information and information containing energy, the yin-yang symbol is a circle showing both yin and yang flowing with each other as well as within each other—to demonstrate their eternal interplay and energetic interdependency. (You'll learn more about this in chapter 5.)

This same "quantum" message of informed power is the medical basis for all of life as conveyed in Ayurveda, naturopathic, homeopathic, and mind-body medicine. In my own experience, all small—and all profound—changes in your performance and life can be orchestrated by connecting with the right energy at the right time.

Informed Power in Everyday Life

Historically, alternative and conventional sciences have always been regional, especially when it comes to techniques and discoveries. This can, on occasion, become a real barrier to anyone trying to access the precise concepts and skills to live the best life they can. Asian holistic medicine and psychology, for example, have been developing energy-enhancing skills and exercises for many years. In addition, there is no shortage of energy-building and -enhancing techniques that have been researched and proven effective by the Western sciences. It is imperative that we combine resources in order to reap the benefits of both, accessing the most effective and progressive set of energy-enhancing, life-building tools possible.

Let's take a look how some effects of informed power can come together in simple, everyday experiences.

Imagine that the phone rings as you are reading this chapter. On the other end is your boss informing you that you are getting an unexpected raise in your salary. Almost immediately, you begin to feel a certain force behind the information your boss is relaying to you. This force may manifest as a surge of excitement, joy, or well-being. It will, however, feel and play out with greater or lesser intensity, sparking different thoughts, emotions, and actions than if you had, say, received a call from a romantic partner expressing their love to you, or a call from a relative announcing that someone close to you has suddenly passed away.

The reason for this is that the informed power in each example will shape and trigger different psychological as well as physiological reactions in your mind and body; and this will, in turn, change the way you are feeling. These feelings can last and infiltrate other things you do during the day and the experiences of other individuals you encounter.

In general, whenever you set out to do something, you need a certain amount of informed power to get the job done. Your goal may be to feel focused for a professional presentation, to fight off insomnia, or to simply have a good day at work. Whatever the case may be, making yourself aware of what kinds of energies are already affecting you and whether you need to change any of these energies will facilitate your goal.

Your ability to successfully reach your goals can increase by how well you match the energy to the situation. The good news is that a little knowledge of the workings of your mind and body will go a long way. For example, consider Lily, who is fifteen and loves techno music. On a day when she was having a test at school, she decided to load up her iPod and listen to dance tunes before she left her home. She played them all the way into school.

Her father, on the other hand, can't stand techno and insisted that her time would be better spent taking one last look at her notes. But Lily told him not to worry, that his getting so emotional—as well as his lack of confidence in her—was more apt to distract her when she took the test than the music she had been playing, which she believed would help. Her response frustrated him all the more.

To her dad's surprise, a few days later Lily came home with an A on her test. Her father regretted the hard time he had given her, but he also had difficulty believing that the music had anything to do with her good grade. Lily, on the other hand, claimed that it was the music that helped her do well. Who was right?

Energy Medicine

Scientifically speaking, sound is a form of energy. Its effects on us are both electrical and chemical. Like all energy, it contains both force and information.

For instance, what you feel when you listen to sound (in Lily's case, techno music) will largely depend on information you already have in your mind—i.e., how much you understand the structure of the song, how much you already like the particular piece, and what parts you like best and anticipate. One person's perfect prescription for high quality energy that will enhance her memory, speed of recall, and ability to concentrate can very well be another person's poison, paralyzing their ability to do any of those things.

Techno worked for Lily because she loves it and understands its structure, so it does not sound like chaos to her, as it does to her father. Consequently, its fast tempo and rhythmic patterns are able to change the pattern of her *brain waves* (electrical currents in the brain). This change then triggers further *electrochemical* changes throughout her, physiologically and psychologically. These multiple interactions generate and strengthen the specific feeling of alertness and readiness she wants for her test. Her feeling that the music altered her mind-set is real, and it can be as effective in terms of energizing her as a prescription drug or a caffeinated drink—with an exception: she can learn to make this effect last longer and even trigger automatically.

Did Lily need to use techno to do well on her test? No, not necessarily, as there were plenty of other energy sources (and even styles of music) from which she could have chosen. But to have sensibly chosen differently, her other option would have had to work just as well—or better—and she would have had to have the desire to discover it.

Techno worked just fine in this case, giving Lily the mental and physical energy she needed. She was satisfied with her mind-set and her grades, so this way of energizing herself before tests was safe, effective, and made sense. Plus, it was fun and easy.

As was discussed earlier in this chapter, your body uses various types of energy, including light, chemical, electric, heat, mechanical, and sound. Tapping into these different everyday energies can help you with daily goals. Not only that, but you can learn to mix your own blends. Using sound—whether it is recorded or imagined—is only one way to do this, and we will explore many others. What's more, you will learn how to strengthen and quicken these energies' desired effects on you, as well as train your mind to seek and connect with them automatically. What's key is learning to first identify your personal energy needs. This is so important that we will spend the whole next chapter on the topic.

Subtle Energies

Subtle energy is a term first introduced to the world of science by physicists David Bohm and Yakir Aharonov in the early 1960s to describe not directly visible and apparently intelligent energy in the body and throughout the environment, which we are beginning to be able to observe with today's powerful imaging instruments. Often referred to as *chi*, *ki*, *prana*, and life force energy, subtle energies are important because they provide verifiable information about energies that affect your life yet are operating at a speed faster than light. Although much more new science on subtle energy and its effects and uses is necessary, and will be advancing in the years ahead, what we currently know about it is cause for significant discussion.

The work done by many prominent scientists like Dr. Richard Davidson, Dr. Masaru Emoto, Dr. Gary Schwartz, Dr. David Bohm, Dr. Yakir Aharonov, and Dr. Deepak Chopra continues to show that these subtle energies can be tapped via physical and mental techniques we already recognize, such as chi kung acupoint stimulation, visualization, and meditation, which have concrete science behind them. Adding these tools to your skill kit will allow you to access the full spectrum of energy available to you.

For some of us, at certain points in our lives, subtle energy may be the only resource to help resolve or support us during troublesome or painful life situations that need management and solution. Skill in enhancing life's subtle energies may provide, for example, a reasonable alternative to long-term chronic-pain management. This is especially good for individuals in situations where conventional pain treatment is working less than 100 percent, or where various treatments conflict and are creating further health problems.

From the perspective of holistic and quantum medicines, subtle energies are essential because they help you know your deepest Self. They also assist you in pursuing and achieving both daily successes and longer range intentions. Furthermore, they can prevent illness (and its damages) before it even occurs by helping you identify and eliminate mismatched energy that stresses and deteriorates your daily operations, physiologically and mentally, detatching you from patterns that will wreak havoc in your life down the line. Elimination of mismatched energies also allows subtle energies to instead attach you to higher, balanced, informed power that will keep you healthier and happier. The ability to use the full spectrum of these energies preventatively and curatively is on the frontier edge of today's medicine and will certainly play a primary role in the future of healthcare.

Energy Management

As mentioned, there are many types of energy available to us; how we mix and match them with daily needs is vital.

In the coming pages, you will find that there are temporary means of getting the energy boost you want. Although they are short term, they can be exactly what you need at the moment. Yet very few—if any—of these quick fixes (like an energy drink) can provide the informed power a halfback needs to explosively break through a tonnage of human linebackers and run the ball to a touchdown, or the informed power a cancer patient needs for spontaneous remission.

Instead, the lasting types of informed power come from other sources, such as sound, light, and a broad band of even subtler frequencies. These sources can electrochemically be formed into new *energy templates* (new circuits) in the mind so that they will not run out like a pill or caffeine or other temporary sources. In fact, they can last forever in some cases if you wish. The following chapters will teach you a variety of ways to do just that.

Exercises and Practices

1. The next time you are setting the dinner table, take a slow breath and pause for a moment. Pay attention to what you are feeling energy-wise. How would you describe the way your energy feels? Are there mixed feelings? If so, what are they? Which of these facilitate what you are doing and which do not? What do you think is responsible for the various energies you are feeling?

2. When you are channel surfing on your television or radio, identify how you feel physically and mentally as you go from one station to another. See if you can identify the information coming at you and any opening up within you that is responsible for the different feelings being sparked. For example, consider if the information you were affected by was connected to something someone said. Was it the sight of a certain character or character type? A certain situation, environment, or sound? Consider which of the "shows" you sampled will help you achieve the informed power you need for what you will be doing next. Which will not?

3. Tomorrow morning, when you wake up, as soon as you put your feet on the floor, start paying attention to how various things you look at and touch make you feel.

4. Words contain information and energy. They work like remote controls on a person's behavior. Consciously see how words and phrases you use throughout the day affect other people. Try out a variety of gentle language on people, noticing what effect it has. Similarly, pay attention when those around you use language that has force, but also pay attention to the message behind the words.

2

IDENTIFYING HOW ENERGY AFFECTS YOUR WHOLE PERSON

We are just like tuning forks,
copying the resonances we "touch" energetically.
—Penney Peirce

From sunrise to sunset, you encounter an enormous flow of energy into and throughout your entire being. This informed power has a range of influences on you throughout the day. Whether you feel it or not, it determines how your day evolves, what works out and how satisfyingly, what doesn't work, and how you generally feel both emotionally and physically.

Several decades ago, I sat in my first martial arts class. My sensei ("teacher" in Japanese) was talking about energy. He told the class that the body is a vessel that can hold only a certain amount of energy. Our job, according to him, was to empty out the bad (or dysfunctional) energy and replenish it with the good. To help us understand what he meant, he taught us a simple breathing exercise. Dating back to the Shaolin monks in 525 AD, these breathing techniques are used to increase concentration and strength.

"First, relax," my sensei said. "But not so much that you lose your concentration."

He told the class to slowly breathe in through their noses and out through their mouths, releasing any stress and negativity they were feeling as they exhaled. This would not only increase our power of focus but our external strength. He told us to visualize our breath as vibrant, white light pulsating with energy. This would clean the body and mind of bad energy and increase the good energy.

My notion of martial arts up until then had been limited to a series of drills and movements that could be used for confidence building, self-defense, and de-stressing. But here was my instructor telling me that concentrating inwardly would increase not only my overall focus but my external strength. I was fascinated.

Sometime after my breathing lesson, I decided to test my sensei's words. I had to stack several cords of wood in preparation for winter. It was an early autumn evening, and the sky was orangish gold, its dimming light flickering on the trees and moist ground in the woods. The air was crisp and cidery and sweetened with the scent of bonfires. I had set a goal of one cord for the night, but it had already been a long day, and I was tired.

With nearly half a cord to go, I humored myself and decided to try out my sensei's breathing technique.

I relaxed. I regulated my breathing, as he had instructed, and visualized my mind and body blazing with vibrant and flowing energy. My labor transformed into a meditation of sorts—not that I thought of it that way; it just happened that way. I seemed to forget about my work, yet I worked spiritedly, continuing the breathing exercise as I went along. Rather than begrudging my work, I felt comforted by it. When I finished, instead of feeling my usual soreness and tiredness, I felt restored and animated. I felt energized and joyful. Not only had I done things with much less effort but I felt generally happy. This exercise caught my attention and marked my first step into a new way thinking and feeling. This would evolve over the years into a quest to understand more about how various energies affect the mind and body, and how they can enhance your experience of life.

The Benefits of Regulated Breathing

Although regulated breathing is a traditional idea, it provides the foundation for many energy-building techniques in the world of psychology, medicine, and holistic medicine. This is why so many wellness programs, whether in the ivory towers of academia or in a tiny yoga class in your hometown, begin with simple breathing techniques. It is also why so many mindfulness exercises, which are currently the rage in Western medicine, begin with the same breathing skills. I wasn't surprised to find that associates from Harvard and Columbia Universities, with whom I worked on collaborative projects, used these techniques effectively as part of their clinical work.

But how can a breathing technique turn an everyday chore into an energy-building activity rather than an energy-consuming activity?

From a scientific perspective, better breathing is a good first step toward calming your body and mind and reversing the effects of stress. We know that stress can contribute to poor focus, depression, diabetes, and many other health concerns. But with stressors out of the picture, you will be stronger and healthier, and you will perform better. Furthermore, once you're calm, the positive energy you tap can come on more quickly and smoothly, and will last longer. So as my sensei suggested, it is good to empty your mind and body of stressful energy and replace it with something better.

In terms of overall energy, measured breathing works like a good self-massage. When you breathe in, your diaphragm descends, massaging your abdominal organs, and your lungs expand. As you breathe out, your diaphragm massages back again against your lungs, helping them to expel carbon dioxide. The activity is like a gentle, internal rubdown that opens various acupoints within the body and releases your natural energy flow.

The sound of your breath causes a *functional* (positive) *distraction* (much like music did for Lily). This distraction enables your mind to be smoothly launched from where it is at the moment into a new place as well as a new *frequency* that, with practice, becomes associated with calm yet heightened energy. The sound and association, in turn, are literally (and naturally) able to change the pattern of your brain waves.

Such changes are similar to what can be generated electronically with a *neurofeedback device*. These devices prompt the brain to release a cascade of chemical changes into the bloodstream, which, in my case, alerted, calmed, and strengthened me, supplying me with the mind-set and quality of focus I needed to successfully complete my job. These brain-produced chemicals are so powerful that a healthcare provider would need a license to dispense a commercial version.

More than anything, though, using this simple, regulated breathing exercise helped me to tap all areas of the body's energy resources—light, chemical, electrical, heat, mechanical, sound. It simultaneously soothed and energized me, ultimately making me feel euphoric—a combination of sensations I registered (and ingrained) in my mind as joy.

Finally, regulated breathing—because of its capacity to focus you in the present as well as immediately connect your mind and body—can be extremely useful in preparing you to detect and interact with the more subtle energies.

Increasing Your Sensitivity

The Chopra Center Mind-Body Medical Group writes, "Even though the body appears to be a material object, in reality it is a field of energy, transformation, and intelligence. When we look beyond the molecules that make up the matter of the body, we see fields of energy."[1] Again, moving faster than the speed of light, these subtle energies give you further perspective into the energetic operation of your full living being of body, mind, and spirit.

Most of us experience subtler energies unconsciously. But as you become more sensitive to a fuller spectrum of energies within your personal world and gain a few new tools, you will be able to identify and make use of not only the more obvious energies influencing you but also the less obvious ones. You'll find, incidentally, that the subtle influences—the temperature of the air around you or a certain thought or emotion—are no less effective and often more powerful.

Making yourself more sensitive will help you discern and amplify a wide range of specific effects that, in turn, enable you to determine how you want to be feeling. From there, you can literally build a new brain, with new brain circuits to keep you balanced and flowing, physically and mentally, from one daily situation to another. And this will cause a chain reaction, bringing greater positivity to other things you do because you're feeling better.

Many people begin their day with some kind of nutrition, exercise, or ritual that makes them feel good right off the bat. Wanting to feel this way is natural, as it is your desire to be able to fire up, focus, and feel strong during the day and then relax later into a nice evening and a good night's sleep.

Like most people, you probably already have a natural inclination toward some of these desires already. These tendencies are helpful because you can build off of them, training your mind to automatically tap and issue the specific energy you want, as well as give you a larger, longer-lasting dose of this energy as needed. If a healthy morning routine is not your way at the moment, don't worry. There are many activities you can choose from to get you started.

TRY THIS!

Take a moment right now to let your eyes focus on a few different objects in your immediate field of vision. This information is streaming into your mind at eleven million bits per second and triggering a myriad of electrical and biological responses within you. Although you can focus on only forty bits maximum, you can broaden your receiving band and just experience the myriad of changes you feel, without thinking about or focusing on any particular piece of information. Do this even though, as you peer from one object to another, you may "feel" one to be more relaxing and soothing, busy or distracting, or perhaps irritating or disturbing. Try making yourself more sensitive to (feel into) the stream of data. You may experience sensations of warmth or tingling as the information passes through your mind and body. With a little practice, you can feel electrical and even hormonal changes streaming through you.

What's Happening Under Your Radar?

Some of your energy events will be short lived; others can run for longer periods of time, and sometimes even stay with you for life. Some may be obvious to you, subtle, or may run totally under your radar. Individuals suffering from post-traumatic stress disorder (PTSD), for example, often feel the effects of an energy event for years, and many will feel these effects for life.

But an energy event doesn't have to be "loud" to have staying power. Subtle exchanges have that too. A young child noticing a parent's look of disapproval or disgust can affect the way she sees life, socializes, feels, and thinks for years. From a psychological perspective, you can trace many adult tendencies (good and bad) back to subtle, early-childhood energetic events. In contrast, a song you listened to with your mom or dad in the warm and safe comfort of their arms can shower your life with long-term balance and joy. We know some hardwired reasons why this is true, and we will discuss these as we progress.

Your energy, like everyone's, is flowing and changing from one minute to the next. Whether much of this is happening unconsciously or not, it means that, ultimately, you don't ever have to feel energetically stuck. You have a choice in how you want to be.

Part of that choice is making yourself more aware. This is a hallmark of all holistic medicine and arts. Remember your job is "to empty out the bad (or dysfunctional) energy and replenish it with the good." You choose to get rid of the harmful energies you carry inside, keep any incoming harmful energies at bay, and increase your positive and useful energies. Most important, you increase your mindfulness so that the energy you operate with (your informed power)—the energy you are—comes and grows with your approval. Philosophically, because this informed power that is "you" is also capable of sending out information and then affecting and changing everything it touches, its positive and creative cultivation is your gift to the Universe, as well as your way of making a difference within your life, family, community, and beyond. And with that comes responsibility, as well as deeper personal joy.

Assessing Your Incoming Energy

A college student is heading to class to take a test when she casually bumps into a classmate who talks to her about the exam. He veers off topic for a few seconds, randomly mentioning the class presentation she gave the other day was "creative." That word, creative, makes her momentarily feel good, and then, without skipping a beat, the conversation goes back to their main focus—the test. She takes the test and later finds she received an A+.

Most students won't connect their performance on a test to something that happened unconsciously in their mind beforehand. This is because our energy "downloads" are often unconscious yet in sync with our goals, so we ignore them and attribute success to some other factor.

On the other hand, when things aren't working out, we tend to start looking for reasons why. Oftentimes, the greater a person's problems, the greater his or her concern over what caused them.

Imagine, for a moment, a business professional (let's call him Bob) who is headed into a meeting with the CEO of his company whose support he needs to acquire a contract for a new product he really wants to carry. While standing outside the meeting room, a colleague shows Bob a magazine cover he has downloaded on his cell phone. It pictures supermodels (male and female) in lush vacation spots that are very different from the city where Bob and his employment are currently located. Bob comments on how much fun the models appear to be having in such a dream location.

In just milliseconds, Bob's mind-set can change. In fact, this happens so fast (fires in his brain at a speed of around one eight-hundredth of a second) he isn't even aware of it. Where the lack of exoticness in his own life was of no issue just seconds before, it subconsciously bothers him now. The paradise presented by the magazine cover has caused his life to suddenly look and feel drab in comparison. The effects of this unconscious bias manifest during the meeting: Bob now feels negative about his own life situation, which causes him to lose focus, forget important details, and appear disorganized. He feels as though his mind has a mind of its own. And in a way, it does. This subtle feeling is an indication that something in the meeting may go awry.

Once such feelings of disorder bubble up into your field of awareness, what you do next is important—at least as significant as your imminent goals. You can shrug them off and let them pass like water under the proverbial bridge until you literally forget they ever happened. Or you can trace them to their source, defining what energy sparked your reaction (in Bob's case, bias and loss of control).

If I showed you a video clip of Bob's meeting, you would see external signs of Bob's interest in the pictures on his colleague's cell phone. Bob might even comment, if he himself were watching the video, that he has no problem liking what the pictures show. Yet later, as the all-important meeting proceeds, you would see (and perhaps hear) Bob's physical and psychic energy at a deficit. The essential energy he needs to keep him alert, focused, and better able to reason things out would elude him.

It may not seem possible that a picture on a cell phone could so completely derail someone's day, but such phenomena can and do happen all the time. The key to dealing with such situations when they happen to you is to become aware of them. For example, if you think, *My mind seems to have a mind of its own*, that's always a good signal that one of these situations is occurring.

This subtle awareness is energetically coming from what some might call your *consciousness*, or what we in mind-body medicine (as well as those in various philosophies of enlightenment, such as Buddhism and Taoism) call your *higher mind* and *highest* (spiritual) *mind.*

In mind-body medicine, the mind is both *local* and *nonlocal.* Your local mind is associated with your body and the brain's networks. This is referred to as the *physical mind*, or *lower mind.* The next "step up" is your *higher mind*, associated with *nonlocal consciousness* (outside the body), and third is your highest mind, which is associated with your spirit (nondenominational).

In mind-body medicine, "mindfulness" is everything because it allows you access to your being's full energy system. Mindfulness can place your awareness at all three levels. And although most people will begin to explore mindfulness in the lower mind, with practice, we all can move our way up and within all three levels simultaneously.

I use the term *tri-level consciousness* to refer to full-being mindfulness. Though it would not be desirable to attempt to operate with tri-level consciousness all the time, there are times when you absolutely need it. You will discover in the coming pages how to identify these moments when tri-level consciousness is needed. You will also learn techniques that will enable you to activate all three levels of consciousness; and you will learn about what powerful physical, mental, and spiritual successes this open-energy highway can trigger.

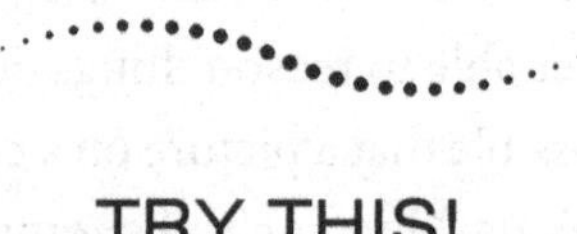

TRY THIS!

Just pick any neutral object in the environment you are now in. Take a few relaxed breaths and focus on that object. Try to keep your mind totally neutral—no thoughts, no feelings, no images. Remain focused on your chosen object for several minutes. See if any thoughts, feelings, or images start popping into your field of concentration. This will give you an idea how your mind is functioning; for example, it might be relaxed or jumping quickly from topic to topic. It will also give you a glimpse into what may be influencing your mind at any given moment. Then imagine a light switch capable of turning these influencers off. Now go ahead and turn them off one at a time, using your switch. When the distractors return, turn them off again. When you do this, you are using your higher mind to teach your brain—your local mind—how you want it to operate.

Practice this activity periodically until your mind gets the message that you want these distractors turned off; you want your mind clear.

The more you practice turning off those elements, the easier it becomes, and the longer you can sustain an unaffected mind-set.

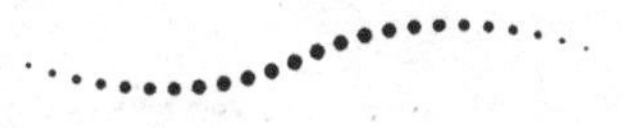

Influence and Energy

Trial attorneys are well acquainted with energetically guiding another individual's mind without that person being aware of what is happening. A certain video, picture, or word delivered in a way that a juror may perceive as random can have instant swaying and powerful effects. This is because pictures, words, gestures, and so on are themselves made of informed power that can be copy-pasted into a juror's mind and body. Such prompts carry with them the informed power to sway people's opinions one way or another. We take in and send out such energy—mostly unconsciously—all the time.

From a scientific perspective, the luxurious pictures Bob's colleague innocently showed him set off an electrochemical response in Bob's brain—which then issued a cascade of hormones that depressed his overall mental and physical state. If afterward, you were to ask Bob if the picture on the cell phone had anything to do with his performance in the meeting, he (like most people) would very likely say no.

This is why your first job is to become aware.

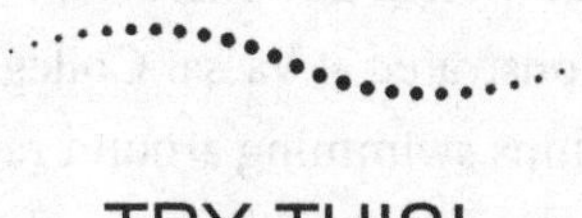

TRY THIS!

The next time someone compliments you, pay attention to how it makes you feel. Be specific with your descriptors. Does the compliment drive your energy up, make you self-conscious, or increase your confidence? Later on, see if you can trace those feelings and how they may have energetically influenced the way you operated in the situations that followed.

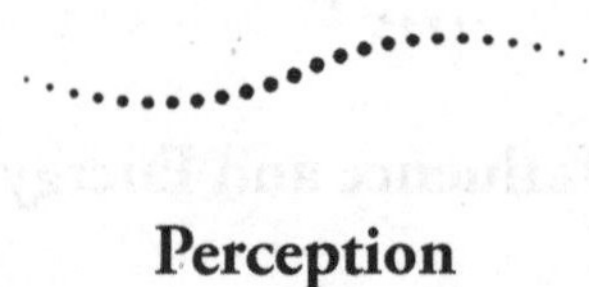

Perception

As you become more sensitive to how various energies you encounter are influencing you, you will also need to become mindful of how you perceive these elements.

Perception is the process of organizing and interpreting information. It includes sensory information received from the five senses: touch, sight, smell, hearing, and taste. It also involves the cognitive process of recognition, which is triggered by the sum of your experiences. For example, you recognize a certain scent as lemon because you "know" what lemon is; or you recognize a certain face as Maria Smith's because you know who Maria Smith is. A person who is unfamiliar with the English language and doesn't know what the word "creative" means won't have much of a response to someone complimenting him as such. Or if the only experiential context you have for the term *creative* is when it means you are doing things inappropriately (as in "creative accounting"), you would have a totally different response.

A well-known illustration of how important experience is in our perception of life was demonstrated at Vassar College in 2007.[2] Pictured in a vase is a group of dolphins swimming around randomly. When viewing the picture, however, most adults will not see the dolphins—at least not at first. Instead, they will perceive that in the vase is an image of two adults, a man and a woman, embraced intimately. Affected by what you already know and have experienced in life, you may see something quite different. It has been reported, for example, that when presented with the same picture, children almost always see the dolphins and entirely miss seeing the two intimately embraced adults—even when they are told to look for them. The reason is that most children have not experienced such details of adult intimacy.

Sometimes one or more of an individual's senses may be deficient. Such a situation can play tricks on your perception. For instance, individuals who have experienced severe burns may lose varying degrees of tactile sensitivity. One burn victim I know cannot sense when heat sources may be too hot and, as a result, needs to be especially vigilant.

Perceptions can begin as personal and then go viral, so to speak. As an example, introverts are commonly misunderstood in family, social, and academic environments. This happens because their particular type of energy is not within the observer's world of conscious experiences and, as such, is often unidentifiable. So "compensation"—behavior emerging from a conscious or unconscious drive to offset a real or imagined deficiency through the observer's reaching a more balanced view and response—is not likely to happen.

I recently witnessed an academic institution giving a workshop on how to "change" the introverted student, a proposal that was obviously based on the perception and assumption that all introversion is the same and that change is what such an individual must need. It is so easy for a teacher to conclude, for instance, that the child in the back of the classroom is not interested in or struggling with a particular lesson because the child is silently looking out the window. But the student may simply be thinking over things deeply. In fact, the student may be making deeper connections than those students who appear interested because they are doing all the talking. In such cases, the teacher frequently bases his perceptions on his own former experiences. This perception can be detrimental to his accurate assessment and rapport with the introvert, and with the other students too. It can have a damaging energetic effect that ripples through his classes for weeks—perhaps a whole school year.

How does this affect all the other students to whom the teacher's reactions are being transmitted? Both teacher and students are capable of transmitting this inaccurate mind-set to other individuals, places, and situations they encounter.

As a footnote, I want to gently mention that how we interact with various energies from the world around us and how we loop them forward bears responsibility to a bigger picture, beyond ourselves.

Be Aware of Different Ways of Perceiving

You have a choice in how you perceive events and the world around you. Imagine you are heading out for a jog and just as you hit the play button on your iPod, you realize it is out of power. Instead of getting irritated, you could perceive this as an opportunity to be more attentive to the natural environment. Or say you have come down with the flu right before you are to give a professional presentation and have to reschedule it. Instead of perceiving the flu as an obstacle, you could see it as a way to enhance your PowerPoint with components you didn't have time to explore and develop previously.

This way of seeing information is what I call a *perceptive filter*: information you carry in your memory and draw upon to help you analyze and respond to other information and events. These filters can be good or bad, depending on whether they help you identify and accomplish positive goals or keep you from them. The good news is you can learn to energetically enhance, edit, or short circuit and replace your perceptive filters to make them more effective and appropriate to things you do.

In an ideal situation, you are self-aware of the perceptive filters you are engaging, and you will continue to edit or add to those that are appropriate, rather than giving your mind over to filters that turn currents and chemicals on and off inside you, without your approval.

Use Your Mind's Filtering Mechanism

Being able to phase out certain dysfunctions from your field of consideration improves your energy and performance. This is called *good inhibition*. It allows you to focus on something not because you are narrowing your vision to that one item but because you are excluding everything else you deem irrelevant, so that the real subject of your interest remains crystal clear. Remember, you are not obligated to focus on, pursue, or respond to "stuff" just because it enters your life; nor should you if it is detrimental to you physically, mentally, or spiritually.

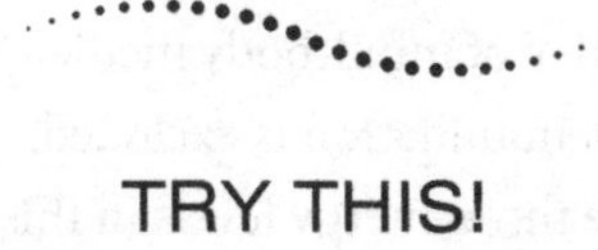

TRY THIS!

The next time you are in a coffee shop or park, scan your surroundings and look for people or things that you are attracted to. Then ask yourself why you find them attractive. Get specific. Is your attraction subtle or more dramatic? Now look for something that sparks negativity in you. Again, try to specifically identify why. Ask yourself what in your world of experience is triggering your feelings and conclusions.

The Three Energy Levels

Imagine that a group of engineers are evaluating an individual's body structure to determine the exact amount of force she can issue if she were to strike a solid block of ice with her fist just once. To accomplish their evaluation, they use a myriad of tests, imaging instruments, and what appear to be complicated algorithms. They scientifically conclude there is no way this specific body can issue enough force to fracture the massive ice block. Then they attach electrodes to her so that data can be sent to a computer screen where they can analyze it. They ask her to strike at the ice. She relaxes, closes her eyes, and takes a deep breath. Then she loudly exhales and sounds a skin-tingling "*Kiai*!"

The ice instantly explodes. Data streams to the computer screen. Somehow, she has issued far greater force than they thought she was anatomically capable of. What just happened?

Let's start by considering the spectrum of energy flowing into your own daily life—energy from your physical world, your mental/emotional worlds, and your spiritual world. Please note: when I use the term *spirit*, I use it from the perspective of mind-body medicine and not as a religious term, and as such, no denomination is excluded.

You can chart these three energy levels in this way:

Spirit (highest mind)
Mind (nonlocal realm of higher mind)
Body (physical realm and local mind)

And if you are thinking that these energy levels correspond to the spectrum of tri-level consciousness we spoke of earlier, you are right—they do.

Each energy level of body, mind, and spirit has different characteristics, but together, they constitute you—the whole you. When you are conscious of all three levels at once, you experience your whole living being. When all three are synchronized and harmonious, you are and feel *unified*.

Each energy level interacts with and can affect the others. Furthermore—and vitally—you can transfer and transform the energy from one energy level to the next. When all you believe in (or perceive) is material or physical-realm energy, then you have a hard time imagining how the martial artist in the above story (or anyone) could exceed the amount of force their physical anatomy is capable of issuing. It is through the transfer and transformation of energy that this becomes possible.

At the energetic level of daily experience, in fact, anyone can learn to exceed the cage of their own physical, cognitive, and emotional limitations to increase energy quality.

The energy you encounter each day is constantly interacting and affecting all three levels of your consciousness. This is important because it means that you can feel (and self-generate) what is called *downward causation*—i.e., you can consciously choose to transfer specific informed power from higher energy levels downward. This downward movement increases your energy and information resources, and most important, can be used to retrain your mind and body to evolve the way they operate to higher levels.

When you do this, your energy both transfers (moves down) and transforms to the next level's frequency. Such energy movement is a two-way street, so each level can extend influence (again, informed power) into the other. You can also move energy upward. You have heard the phrase "mind over matter"; I like to use the phrase "body over mind" to describe this. For example, if your mind glitches (emotionally or contemplatively), you can sometimes benefit from temporarily detaching and engaging in physical exercise for a while, then returning to the task at hand.

In our earlier ice-block example, the woman was able to transfer downward the informed power she needed so that she could shatter the ice with a single strike.

Chart Your Energy Day

As has been mentioned, the various energies you experience during your day come in many forms, including people, emotions, things you read, and foods. These energies influence you and are affected in turn by your perceptions.

Knowing what energies influence you and how they do so can be useful for many reasons. These reasons include being able to identify which energies in your environment support your desires and goals, provide you with strength and endurance, and keep you healthy and in a flowing mind-set. One way to get a good overview of what energies are presently influencing you is to create a table. This will better your ability to mix and match the specific energies you need for daily endeavors and manage or eliminate those that are dysfunctional.

The next page shows a table that tracks how Audrey, a forty-two-year-old business professional, was affected by the energy she encountered during a typical day. Notice how Audrey gets things done more effectively when her energy is more positive.

Self-Evaluate Your Energy Day

Your first job in learning how to regulate your own daily energy is to pay attention to what energies are affecting you and how. Let's look at Audrey's chart as an example.

The first thing Audrey discovered was that she only felt her mind, body, and spirit were balanced twice all day: when she first saw her partner (but then that changed) and when she had lunch. She could, however, remember herself calming and starting to feel more balanced when she visited the coffee shop.

That surprised her because she was unaware that she felt out of balance, though she admits that being unaware did not lessen any of the depleting energy influences. The other surprise was remembering the influence of her partner's initial positive energy. In light of everything that followed, she'd lost track of that.

Audrey's Day	Events and Thoughts	+ Physical Effects	– Physical Effects	+ Mental Effects	– Mental Effects	+ Spiritual Effects	– Spiritual Effects
Wake-up	Still tired, would like to sleep in		Experienced fatigue, muscle soreness		Felt nervous, unsettled		Felt nervous, unsettled
	Encountered partner	Felt more awake, muscle soreness eased, felt balanced		Felt safe, balanced		Felt safe, balanced	
	Fought with partner		Began sweating, had a jumpy stomach		Felt irritated, unbalanced, unhappy, unsafe		Felt irritated, unbalanced, unhappy, unsafe
Morning	Listened to an aggressive/negative radio show on hectic drive into work				Felt irritated, did not feel balanced		Did not feel any; effects were unavailable or blocked
	Thought about being late		Experienced redness on face		Felt stressed		Felt blocked
	Visited a coffee shop on the way to work			Felt calmer, experienced increased focus and positivity		Felt more balanced; blocks seemed to be dissolving	
Lunch	Ate lunch at the office	Felt tension mildly decrease, felt balanced		Experienced increased psychic energy, felt balanced		Felt mildly happy, balanced	
Afternoon	Checked Twitter and saw I lost two followers		Felt fatigued, muscle tightness		Felt irritated and discontent, loss of focus, declining motivation		Did not feel any; effects were unavailable or blocked
	Took a short coffee break	Had a brief, low-quality bump in physical energy	Experienced increased muscle tightness	Had a low-quality bump in mental acuity	Experienced weak mental focus and low motivation		Felt blocked
	Checked the Dow and saw that it was up for the day	Experienced a mild, momentary energy spike		Felt minimally calm, focused	Did not feel calm or focused enough to feel balanced		Felt blocked
Evening	Returned home	Felt a mild decrease in physical tension		Experienced a mild increase in psychic energy	Felt mental fatigue set in as the psychic energy quickly faded		Felt blocked
Bedtime	Had trouble getting to sleep		Felt anxiously awake		Had progressively less psychic energy and focus		Felt blocked
	Woke up at 3 AM and read an email that would need to be dealt with in the morning		Felt awake but tired		Experienced depression		Did not feel any; effects were unavailable or blocked

Audrey recalls, however, that the burst of positive energy she felt when she first encountered her partner was interrupted by negative energy influencers that messed with her head (and work) all day. Could her negative exchanges with her partner have predisposed her for other forms of negativity? Absolutely. Energy exchanges like that, left uncontrolled, can cloak your perceptive lens, contaminating everything else you do.

On the other hand, Audrey discovered that just seeing her partner made her feel happy and spiked her positive energy. This positive spike is one of the reasons she was attracted to him in the first place. By recalling her original energetic attraction to him, such informed power can remain accessible, and be quite soothing and engaging for Audrey (as it can be for all of us who experience something similar with our partners).

Yet, looking over her chart and putting herself back into the incident, she recalls that it only took an instant for her to get angry with him that morning and for her whole body to tense, effectively turning off the positive energy she felt. The negative effects of this encounter then extended throughout the day.

She did, however, find that a little thing like going to the coffee shop at the beginning of her day had an extended "good" energetic effect. But is her feeling real? We'll see in just a moment.

Audrey took note of how often she checked her Twitter account, and she noticed that she couldn't resist checking how the stock market is doing. She notes the rising Dow Jones Industrial Average had a positive effect on her though only slightly and momentarily. She hadn't noticed before that this specific "good vibe" didn't last long. Now she sees it more like a game of Russian roulette; she can see it interrupts any flow she may be experiencing. She also realizes that she fatigues more easily as a result, can't sustain the pleasure (when there is some), starts feeling less flexible, and tasks become more cumbersome. She thinks the fleeting perks are not energetically worth it and wonders what else she does during the day that drains her good energy like that.

Most important, Audrey realizes that her spirit is blocked most of the day, cutting off its positive downward causation—her highest quality energy resource. This means she is unable to receive its vibrantly informed power to help energize and organize her day. Additionally, this blockage doesn't allow her the energy transfer she needs to optimize her physical, cognitive, and emotional activity throughout the day. Instead of cultivating the higher quality energy she needs, she keeps consuming energy without any replenishment.

Related to this, she also sees something unexpected: when she is calm, not in her "do-do-do" mode, all positive elements in her spectrum experience some higher quality energy. This is true even when she goes to the coffee shop on her way to work. However, as she continues to consume coffee throughout the day, she notes its positive effects decline, and its aftereffects contribute to her fatigue and weakening concentration and motivation. Audrey concludes that she is running on low quality energy for most of the day. Further, she cannot keep consuming energy 24/7 without recharging along the way. She also realizes that for much of her day, she operates with mismatched energies that she must learn to manage or eliminate by reducing her attraction to them.

She needs to better match available energies to support both her endeavors and a positive mind-set. To do this, she will need to mindfully access the informed power of her full energy spectrum.

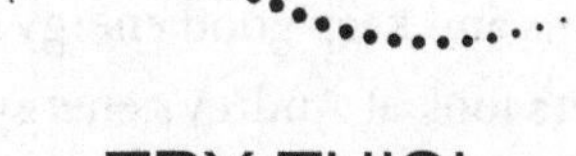

TRY THIS!

Make your own energy table showing the spectrum of things that increase your positive energy and those that decrease your energy or affect it negatively throughout the day. You may want your chart to be more (or less) inclusive than Audrey's chart.

Then, using Audrey's narrative as an example, write a diagnostic narrative based on your own table. See if you can identify how various energies you encounter extend their influence over you. (We'll talk more about energy narratives in the next chapter.)

Experiment by tracking just one item that influences you. Trail it across different situations or times of day to get a clearer assessment of its overall influence on you.

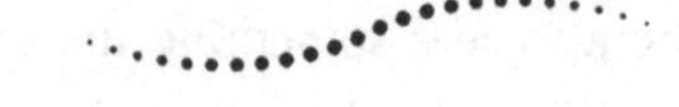

What's *Your* Energy Trap?

An energy drain is anything that depletes your energy. For example, you might find that speaking with a specific person or taking a certain medicine on a particular day drains you of the energy you need for that day. An energy drain may be a one-time thing or it may evolve into an *energy trap*. Energy traps are patterns you have developed (or are developing) that take away your positive energy and mess up your daily activities. An energy trap can also be a situationally specific pattern—for instance, maybe you take a drink of alcohol (or an energy drink) every time you have an issue that requires careful consideration. But the negative effects of these drinks are numerous and include fatigue, lack of creativity, and serious health conditions. Make yourself aware of your energy traps so you can plug these drains and keep good energy flowing.

To illustrate this, let's look at Audrey's energy traps. Like most of us, she has several. Hers are:

- Anger—she experiences toward her partner
- The radio
- Coffee (more than just one morning coffee, as well as an afternoon coffee break)

- The internet (checking Twitter and the Dow)
- Negative thoughts (related to timeliness)

Notice her energy use throughout the day is almost entirely what we refer to as a type A personality or left-brain stuff. This is a high-stress, draining way to go. And it can become a dangerous trap because it is energy consuming and shuts off your energy pipelines of higher mind and spirit. Notice, too, that Audrey does very little to rebuild her energy reserves. This all contributes to her fatigue and irritability and traps her there without relief. When this type of pattern snowballs, it is detrimental to your overall physical and mental health, as well as your feelings of flow and purpose.

Like Audrey, we all have energy traps. The good news is that we have plenty of enjoyable, energy-building options. In the next chapter, we will examine your personal daily energy needs and take a look at some quick and easy tools with which you can meet them. You'll be able to use your new tools to plug and eliminate your own energy drains, and replace those drains with fun, easy, and free energy gains!

Exercises and Practices

1. Randomly check in on your breathing throughout the day. You are almost sure to discover that your breaths are shallow. Relax, slow down your breathing, and breathe deeper. Imagine pulling the air into your lungs starting from the bottom of your lungs up. This will help you breathe more abdominally and with less stress. Count "one" as you breathe in, then again as you breathe out. Repeat this process, adding the numbers two, three, and four. Don't go higher than four. Then start again. Repeat this process for as long as you are comfortable, but not for more than a few minutes at first. Pay attention to how this makes you feel. Name that emotion so you can use it in

specific situations later when you may feel it is in deficiency, or when you feel that summoning it will energetically support a situationally specific task.

2. Call two different people and see how each makes you feel. Look for nuances in how they affect your energy, both short term and longer. Be specific about what those nuances are.

3. The next time someone says something to you and you feel a jolt of negativity or positivity, ask yourself what just happened in your mind? Be specific. Can you identify why you are feeling this way? Ask yourself what reaction you would choose to have in the future.

4. Turn on your television and channel surf. Identify your initial feelings as each show comes up. This will help you practice becoming more sensitive to how various energies affect you.

5. Plant something outdoors if possible. If not, pot a plant indoors. How does this make you feel? Be specific. What are the short-term and long-term effects that this activity has on you?

6. Listen to several pieces of music that you like at home. Think about how each song makes you feel. Make a playlist and listen to it while taking a drive that is relaxing to you. See if your reaction to each song is the same as when you listened to it at home or if your feelings have changed somewhat. Music does not necessarily affect individuals the same way at various times of day or in different environments. See if your reactions change during the day, or when you drive to a significantly different location, or when you start a new task to elicit the most positive effect.

3

IDENTIFYING YOUR ENERGY NEEDS

There's something about taking a plow
and breaking new ground. It gives you energy.

—KEN KESEY

Everyone has different energy needs, but one thing we all have in common is that our minds have the inborn capacity to naturally gather the precise informed power we require for a vivid and brilliantly lived life. Not only that, but the more we use this gift—and the more of us who do—the smoother and more positive life becomes. We set into motion a loop of energy that will optimize our collective (and individual) evolution physically, emotionally, and spiritually. By changing our personal energy, we change the world's energy; and by changing the world's energy, we change our own. This evolution is, in fact, a core mission of *Body Intelligence.*

In order to help you locate and plug into the energy you think you need, your mind creates templates or patterns that kick in automatically, and in milliseconds, *voila*—you're plugged in. As a result of this automatic process, much of the great energy you experience—as well as the fatigue, loss of focus, and disorganization you may feel, within any given day—is self-induced, though not necessarily consciously regulated. This is important to note because, with a little effort, you can deliberately regulate these energies to create an automatic template that will get your mind working to produce the feelings and actions that are authentic to your true character and goals.

What Energy Do You Think You Need?

Tracking how many good and bad vibes you feel in a day can be a real eye-opener. This is because most of these results are connected to the right (or wrong) mix of energy. Once you map them, you can begin to better control them.

Imagine, for a moment, that it is early morning and you have not yet prepared for your day. Still in pj's, you turn on your computer. You begin working on a personal financial concern that's a little thorny, but you feel you can resolve it before heading off to work.

Next thing you know, you've been glued to the computer for nearly two hours (so easy to do!). With only a cup of coffee to hold you over, you perceive your financial problem still looming over you like a dark cloud.

You look at your watch and realize you have a business appointment coming up later in the morning. You get a little anxious but work a bit more without success, finally telling yourself you have to stop or you'll be late for your appointment. You reluctantly turn off the computer and get breakfast.

As you eat, you think about your finances but not so much that it gets in the way of enjoying your meal. Remember, pleasure is a form of energy too, and it is one of the strongest drives. Your choice to have breakfast makes sense because you feel a little more human again, a little more energized, and a little less stressed.

When you finish eating, you lay out nice clothes for yourself and decide on a shower. The expectation of feeling good amidst the refreshing water and dressing your best starts making you feel better already.

Then, as if out of nowhere, as the warm water cascades across your closed eyes, you have an epiphany—what some call a Zen moment. There you are in the shower, having momentarily relaxed and forgotten about everything, and suddenly the solution to your financial conundrum just pops into your head.

Most of us (probably *all* of us) have experienced Zen times when life delivers solutions like this. Although the places of such moments may vary, they come to us similarly. That is, one minute you're wracking your brain, looking for a needle in the proverbial haystack, then, without any effort or warning, the solution is right there on a silver platter. Why does this happen?

One reason is that you have interrupted the concentration process, which, much like a high-wattage appliance, consumes a lot of energy and will eventually leave you drained. By recharging your reserves with good nutrition (chemical energy) and calming yourself down (electrical and chemical energy), you have reversed your fatigue and anxiety and feel restored.

Note, however, that although you feel your mind is idle during such moments, this is only an illusion. We may feel like we are luxuriating in comfort, but our brains are still sparking away in search mode behind the scenes—kind of like the flashlight icon that appears on your computer screen, searching through mounds of data as you mentally take a break and do something fun.

If you could see into your brain during this search, you would see the same areas that had activated earlier, while you were consciously working on your finances, are still active and mining through information for you—only subconsciously and without stress. Next thing you know, refueled by the relaxing shower, your brain has located what you're looking for, and it feels like it has just popped up out of nowhere in your mind.

Here's the take-away point: this process can be self-induced to make problem solving less stressful and, in fact, more pleasurable. In the coming pages, you will learn a wide range of ways to get the process of refueling while your brain mines information working for you. What's more, with repetition, you can train your mind to generate a template that will stream into this mode to refuel you automatically and as needed.

There is another take-away point you may be wondering about: Could this or any epiphany have been induced nonlocally? That is, rather than originating in the physical networks of your brain, could the answer to your financial issue have come from the subtler energy of your higher mind, which is not part of the physical you? From the perspective of holistic medicines, the answer to this question is also yes. In the coming chapters you will learn how to tell the difference between these two forms of consciousness.

Making an Energy Chart

The table on the next page is an energy chart kept by someone I know. His name is Alex, he is thirty-six years old, and he works as a realtor. Alex's table serves as an example for how you can chart your own energy patterns, see how they affect you, and discover what you will need to do to better match the energy you bring into your life with your daily and long-term goals.

In the chart, Alex indicates what type of energy he feels he needs more of as a typical day progresses. Note: he did not mark any time frame as being "perfect as is," which would have indicated that he had the exact energy he felt he needed in that moment.

Following this table is his written *energy narrative.* This narrative helps Alex (and you) trace how the manner in which Alex energizes for one situation affects what happens to him later. An energy narrative can also help you to more accurately understand and track the longer-range effects of your own energy choices. Let's take a look.

Alex's Energy Needs

	Wake-up	Drive to Work	Entering Work-place	Morning	Midday	Afternoon	Drive Home	Evening	Night
Perfect As Is									
High Energy	X	X		X	X	X			
Medium Energy							X		
Low Energy			X					X	X

Note: The table above shows what type of energy Alex feels he needs throughout the day. It indicates that he feels his energy is too low for most of the day, as he is looking for higher energy to sustain him—with exception to his drive home and in the evening, during which times he feels his energy is too high.

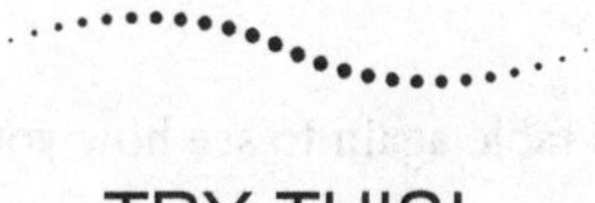

TRY THIS!

Modeling Alex's table, chart your own energy needs as you move through a typical day. Put an X next to the type of energy you feel you need at each checkpoint. If you think the energy you are feeling is perfectly matched to the situation, then check "Perfect as is."

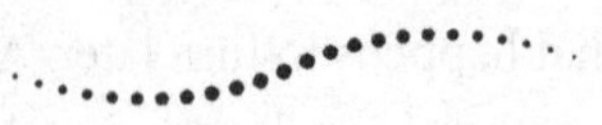

Writing an Energy Narrative

After you make your own energy chart, describing your day in narrative (story) format will give you a more refined perspective on how your energy matches your needs.

Remember, energy is comprised of force and information—in other words, informed power. Typically, a myriad of forces and information affect you simultaneously. As your day progresses from one task to another, you may feel moved by one single informed power, and that power may be going up or down. When you interact with others, the environment, or yourself with more introspection and self-reflection, you can operate with a wider bandwidth. This allows you to monitor a spectrum of energies (channels) simultaneously. You can also identify with specificity what is informing and powering you, whether this influence is functional or not, and how forceful each particular energy is. From here, you can "clean up": eliminate negative influencers (especially the strong ones) and better match up the positive ones with your goals and desires. This is best done in specific situations. Your energy narrative can give you this broader perspective, and help you see that your thoughts, feelings, and actions are a sum total of a number of forces and information.

Let's look at Alex's table again to see how you might write and analyze your own energy narrative.

Consider How You Wake Up

Everybody needs to start off their day in a manner that snowballs positive energy that will get them through their routines. So, a good place to begin your own energy narrative is by first noting how you feel as you wake up and then noting the things you do to get your day in progress.

In his narrative, Alex writes that his first thoughts upon waking are that he feels like pulling the blanket back over his head and sleeping another hour, if not two; he's just not ready to do anything yet. He says it usually takes him about twenty minutes to drag himself out of bed. Alex's unwillingness to wake up isn't just because he went to bed late the night before. His reluctance has become a pattern—the usual. Once a pattern like this is ingrained in your body-mind-spirit, it energetically activates in advance—in this case before Alex even wakes up. His tiredness is an indicator of the influence of mismatched energies.

Getting Ready to Get Out of the House

When he finally gets up, Alex reports that he turns on the television in his bedroom and goes right for the news. It is winter, and he catches himself hoping for a wicked snowstorm so that he can come home from the office early. He says that hearing a forecast of sunny makes him feel worse. His energy declines and his mind-set turns negative, then attracts more like energy.

Following the weather is a national news show, which Alex also finds irritating. But Alex doesn't turn the television off, thinking that hearing the early morning chatter will help wake him up. What Alex is discovering, however, is that the type of conversation he is listening to (and energetically connecting with) on the news has an impact on how his energy evolves. The energy he is listening in on and copying into his own mind and body spikes his brain-wave activity with higher frequencies, so you can see how he thinks it might help him wake up. He perceives its information, however, as negative. Thus, although the news drags Alex out of his slumbering mind-set, rather than generating a joyful mind, the information it carries begins to stress him out. This stressful energy has extended effects that cause Alex to feel disorganized and sluggish throughout the day. Additionally, waking this way regularly will ingrain a pattern that kicks in automatically. After a while, he won't need the triggers. He will wake up irritated automatically. His mind will psychologically and biologically orchestrate it all for him.

Alex downs two large cups of strong coffee and eats a high-protein bar, all on the run, before leaving the house. He is craving clean, robust energy, but it's not happening. Instead of feeling about 80 percent more energetic than when he awoke—which is where he'd like to be—he is feeling about 20 percent.

Alex continues to feel the effects of this mismatched energy pattern. When he gets outside, he remembers he forgot his cell phone in the house. So he races back in to get it and realizes he also left his house and car keys inside too. He thinks, "What's the matter with me?" Feeling like his game is off lowers his available energy even further.

Sound familiar? The problem is that we are all capable of similar days. Many influences—cultural, social, educational—shape our responses to incidents we encounter throughout the day. Some of these influencers are good for us, some bad, and we carry them inside us, mostly at an unconscious level. What's important to know is that you can become aware of these influencers and the energy patterns they establish in you, and you can change all this fairly easily as you need.

The Drive to Work

Alex writes in his narrative that he drives to work. The first thing he does in the car is play aggressive music with bawdy lyrics. He launches himself out of the driveway under this influence. He figures these songs get him excited when he goes out with friends, so why wouldn't they help him rally on his way into work? But they don't. What he really needs is energy that will pick him up physically and simultaneously deliver a calm and vibrant clear-headedness. He is now noticing that, while the songs he has selected fire him up, they also make him feel anxious.

He further realizes the coffee and protein bar he had for breakfast don't settle very well, giving him indigestion. So he takes antacids—twice the recommended dose, he notes—"just to make sure." It occurs to him while writing his energy narrative that the antacids do work (for the time being), but more important, he becomes aware that he doesn't like taking them. He puts some thought into this reaction and discovers that he enjoys seeing himself as athletic but hasn't been able to get out much this winter, because it has been extra cold. He's already a little depressed about being off schedule with outdoor exercise, so taking the pills energetically rocks his self-esteem with the informed power to depress him further and lead to more stress. Seems like a little thing, but to Alex it's not. He feels like his fitness and general health is in decline. This additional negativity drives his available energy further downward and his fatigue and anxiety up. He discovers that this lower energy pattern is what he carries into work. Lacking the calm alertness he really needs makes it more difficult to reverse the negative energy cycle he is caught in.

Entering the Workplace

The way you energetically enter your workplace is very telling. This is the pattern that will unconsciously shape the next things that you do. It is also the way in which you will deal with unexpected situations that cross your path.

When Alex arrives at work, he realizes he feels low and jumpy—what he refers to as "spit on a griddle." Right off the bat, he receives an unexpected email from a frustrated a client. Because Alex's energy is already in a weakened and negative spin, this spikes his anxieties. He nevertheless emails back, but it takes longer than he'd hoped, swinging his mood further downward.

Alex then finds himself addressing several other issues he didn't see coming. When he looks over his narrative, he sees how he progressively becomes more inflexible and irritable through the day. What he needs, he realizes, is a way to regularly decompress his stressors and restore his energy, which appears to be depleting almost all day long. This is a significant realization because, in order to give yourself the energy you need, you have to realize (1) what your exact need is and (2) what energy you are currently plugged into that is not working.

The more effort Alex puts into his daily tasks, he now observes, the more difficult these tasks often seem. He eventually feels disorganized and trapped in a pressure cooker, with no way out. If Alex doesn't change the energy he is cultivating and the templates triggering him, he will keep accruing similar results. But he needs to see that what he does matters. The devil, however, is in the details. Becoming aware of the things you do that give you the right energy for specific tasks and then matching these energies will help put you in charge.

Midday

Some people take lunch breaks and others like to work straight through, or with minimal time off. But everyone needs downtime. Without it, you will deplete your energy. It's important to take a break, live into your energy dips, feel them, and use them to recharge. As noted earlier, your mind can get creative during these mellower moments, making all kinds of connections between new and old information. You may inhibit this capability if you keep barreling forward without downtime. A better choice is to spend this time to fuel your mind's creative mechanism to get it working for you.

As for Alex, still craving more energy, he goes out instead for more coffee. By midafternoon, he is fatigued. He now realizes his affinity for coffee isn't giving him the energy boost he wants, but it would be hard for him to give it up because he likes the respite it offers from his routine.

Could doing something restful during lunch give Alex as much punch as the coffee? The answer is yes—and probably more. In fact, it is by establishing that new kind of pattern that he will find the energy he needs to get him through the rest of the day.

Alex's low and mismatched energy continues to drive him into further problems. Later that day, he bumps into a colleague, loses focus, and talks her ear off about random things. He winds up saying something derogatory about the organization they both work for. It just rolled out of his mouth, and he attributes his lack of control to tiredness. Not a surprise, really, considering the steady mismatch of energies that have driven him from morning till now. His lack of discretion with his colleague then eats away at him periodically for the rest of the day, triggering waves of energy through his mind-body connection that disorganize, stress, fatigue, and depress.

The Drive Home, the Evening, and the Night

Like your drive into work establishes how you enter your workplace as well as affects what ensues once you're there, your drive home can have a similar impact on how you spend your evening.

On his drive home, Alex turns on the radio, hears more op-ed complaining, turns it off, and drives the rest of the way home in silence, feeling the energy fallout of his day. When he gets home, he hits the comfort foods and has a few glasses of wine. Then he promptly falls asleep watching television, wakes up later on, can't get back to sleep, and watches more television in his bedroom until he falls asleep again, around 2:00 AM. It is this kind of mismatched and draining daily-energy pattern that can make you feel stuck.

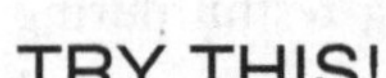

TRY THIS!

Following Alex's example, write your own narrative, being sure to be specific, including both physical and emotional sensations. Your narrative should have a description of how you feel as you first wake up and a description of those things you do in preparing to leave the house after you wake up. Ask yourself about your morning routine. Are your actions motivated by habit or by someone's expectations; or are you consciously choosing such patterns?

Continue the narrative by tracking your energy and its effects as you journey from home to work. Describe what it's like when you get to your workplace; include observations about how your energy affects you.

Also, describe what you do for lunch, giving plenty of detail—especially regarding how the particulars make you feel. Consider whether you are you getting the downtime you need and whether you feel creative during this time. Then track the rest of your day at work. Include your observations about how your energy affects you. Finish your narrative by recording details about your energy for the rest of your day, from the time you leave work to when you go to sleep.

Alex's Energy Traps

As was discussed in connection with Audrey earlier, it is common for many individuals to get caught in energy traps, as Alex has.

Alex's energy traps are:

- Starting his morning by listening to news he doesn't like
- Caffeine—more than one cup in the morning and then adding more to his system later in the day
- Lack of nutritiously balanced meals (too much protein in the morning, low-quality nutrition in the afternoon)
- Car ride to work (with fast, aggressive music and lyrics)
- Use of offensive and derogatory language

You've seen those cartoons where a character gets rolled up, from head to toe, in rope and, consequently, can't move. Each of Alex's energy traps works like another round of rope putting the squeeze on him. The accumulative result of his energy traps is heightened tension, fatigue, loss of motivation and purpose, and sometimes, over excitability. This is a hard regiment of feelings with which to get anything done. In fact, when you operate under these patterns and do manage to generate good results, you often feel like you had to work much harder than necessary, or you get sick or hurt—like the person accidentally hitting his finger with a hammer because his mind and body are under the influence of stressful force and information.

Such energy mismatches can be avoided. But left unattended, they add up and wreak havoc over time.

From the minute Alex wakes up, he feeds his body and mind high, aggressive energy throughout the day—the kind that increases the production of both *adrenaline* and *cortisol* (two stress hormones). The events of his day continue this pattern. He's become an adrenaline junkie, thinking this is what he needs. And this translates into his feeling constricted in mind and body.

Alex cultivates little to no energy with which to balance these effects and loosen up, expand, and flow. Instead, he remains constricted. It doesn't take long for this pattern to become a vicious cycle; many people get caught in such a cycle. If you are feeling this way, you are ready to break out.

Alex is beginning to realize that his intake of energy is mostly the opposite of what he needs. Though he may be groggy when he wakes up, he needs more neutral information than television news can offer. He is partly attracted to the television because (as force) it stimulates his brain-wave activity. Yet, as information, it sends the wrong message, making him stressed.

Caffeine fires the adrenals. No matter how Alex tries to justify it, if he's already stressed and relying on caffeine as his energy fix, it will only add more stress and more exhaustion.

Aggressive language has a similar effect, but let's face it: aggressive words do heighten alertness for certain individuals; we know this.

I recently heard a college football coach laying it on thick to his team to pep them up—to get that little extra elbow grease out of them. When the listener perceives this language in the same way the speaker intends, it will work in the short term, to some extent. Yet this kind of talk, just as the morning news does to Alex, keeps you in a lower energy base by blocking you off from receiving the subtler energies of higher mind, weakening you later, when you really need more strength.

This is a major difference between Eastern and Western thinking and methodology. In traditional martial arts, for example, this kind of aggressive language blocks your access to energies from your higher mind, eliminating the possibility of issuing force beyond your anatomical output. Energy blocks disconnect you from the unity you need in order to use downward causation to transfer the subtler energies through the mind and into explosive biological energy. So, the idea is to keep channels open and avoid the less-productive energies that shut them off. If these energies include certain language, then eliminating that language will work to unblock your energy flow.

In contrast, Phil Jackson, the amazingly successful head coach of the Chicago Bulls, was known for using a different style of aggression: *active encouragement.* Jackson was known as the "Zen Master." The reference characterized his successful use of a different blend of force and information, which was a mix of patience and calm to reduce conflict in and among his players, and to inspire their success.

In our example, Alex's aggressive musical playlist may work to prime him for a night out on the town with his friends, yet it may not be the best choice to enhance his focus on the way to work—especially when he is already irritated and tired. It's not surprising that Alex uses aggressive language later on with his colleague; the energetic pathology for that has been started. Choices he makes all day long add to his unbalanced energy status for that day and can continue to influence him for days ahead—unless he better matches his energy needs with the right juice (power) and the right information.

On the other hand, you can learn to send your mind the messages it needs to recover from irritations. Again, this is as easy as consciously mixing and matching. Methods for achieving this balance are outlined in the following exercises.

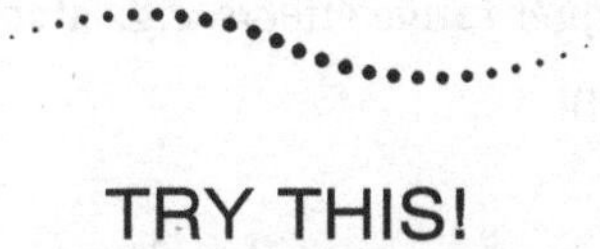

TRY THIS!

Use your narrative to make a list of your own energy traps. Write a detailed commentary about when these traps occur and the circumstances that trigger them.

Exercises and Practices

1. The next time you feel your energy is mismatched for what you are doing, pay attention to how your navigation through that situation also affects subsequent events in your day.

2. The next time you are in the middle of a negative experience (feeling, situation, or thought), ask yourself what you were doing, thinking, and feeling immediately beforehand that may have contributed to destabilizing your energy. Also consider if anyone else was involved.

3. For one day, make yourself aware of the things you do, think, and feel that drain your energy.

4. For one day, make yourself aware of any activities that overstimulate you.

5. List the things in your typical day for which you have a low tolerance. What effect does each have on your overall energy and on you mentally, emotionally, physically, and spiritually? Think in terms of immediate and longer range effects, e.g. later that day, that night, the next day, and so on.

6. The next time someone innocently asks you, "Is something wrong?" just by looking at you, or hearing you say something you thought was neutral, pay attention to your physical state in that moment, especially if the question comes as a surprise. Later on, use a mirror to re-enact your appearance. Try to remember how you looked at the precise moment the comment was made—facial features, posture, and other body movements. See if you can recall anything you were saying—the words you used and your tone. Then, like an actor

might do to get into the mind of a character she is playing, try to re-create it all so you can see what you might have looked like. Ask yourself what details (what energy you were outputting) might have been responsible for your friend's or colleague's impression. Now, use your reflection to practice body and verbal language that you think would have conveyed an impression closer to what you would have liked.

4

USING ENERGY TO BOOST ALERTNESS

When you take your attention into the present moment,
a certain alertness arises. You become more conscious
of what's around you, but also, strangely, a sense of presence
that is both within and without.

—ECKHART TOLLE

Everyone looks for that extra boost of alertness throughout the workday. For many of us, the first place we go is to caffeine, energy drinks, energy bars, or snacks. But there are many other ways to get the lift you want. And if you target these mindfully, using the awareness of your full being or tri-level consciousness, you will more accurately discover and tap the informed power you need. As a result, your actions will be more functionally energized, precise, and balanced.

The amount of stimulation that powers your alertness, however, is not a one-size-fits-all item, so you have to consider your specific tasks or goals. This is because there are different kinds of alertness and different energies that activate them. For example, there is the alertness you want when you wake up in the morning, which is different than the alertness you need to do a difficult math problem or pay attention to a friend or a loved one in conversation. There is the alertness you need to read and analyze a legal document and the kind you use to critique a work of art. There is also the alertness you want to perform an athletic activity and that which you need to stave off (or recover) from serious illness. Most important is the alertness you need to unify the body-mind-spirit connection so that everything you do, decide, and feel consciously comes from the synchronization of your whole and centered Self. When you enter into this state, you and your life flow vibrantly and brilliantly.

As we have been discussing, when you power up more mindfully, you get better at noticing that one type of alertness is not often interchangeable with another. Remember your energy traps? If they are mismatched with the energy you are after, they can leave you fatigued or irritated and send you off course. So again, stepping back and making yourself aware is necessary.

It's not realistic to think that we can be optimally alert 24/7. But as I have said before, we can pick and enhance our alert moments. These moments add up, and with practice, your mind will learn to deliver the precise energy you need automatically. Make a change now, another later, and so on, and your mind and body will sparkle with quality alertness—as needed—in no time.

Psychological Currency

Psychological currency is your bank, so to speak, of psychic (mental) energy. Ranging from lower to higher qualities, it is the informed power you've cached that energizes the mind with positivity, motivation, and the information you need for an activity, feeling, or thought.

Rather than draining you like an energy trap, psychological currency provides you with the necessary force and information to get things done fluidly and happily. The beauty of this mind-set is that when you are in it, your mind is capable of packing more energy than you are consuming, keeping you in the moment, and leaving you energized when you are finished. This is why you can go for hours with what you are doing, losing your sense of time and even place—you are so engaged. And rather than tiring, you feel empowered, lighter, and joyful.

Everyone needs to cultivate and conserve this form of energy; otherwise, doing anything at all becomes laborious at best and impossible at worst. When this energy bank gets low, you need to revitalize it. The good news is that there is a wide range of things you can do to rebalance and hit the road at your best.

I know a waitress at a local diner. Her name is Nancy, and she is consistently pleasant and high spirited whenever I see her there. Once, when I was in the diner, I complimented her on her congeniality. "Here's what keeps me on my toes," she said and opened up her order pad to reveal a photo of her two children. She told me she looks at the picture whenever she needs a little pep. "Keeps me focused and in the right attitude," she said. Just sharing that put a smile on her face.

Sometimes, I can't help but think physiologically. I considered the electrochemical effect of the smile induced by the photo and the calm alertness induced by the higher frequencies Nancy was registering when combined with the pleasurable release of self-produced brain chemicals. I looked at her and thought, *She is certainly in a good zone.* Photos, images, and mentally created imagery are all great ways to add to your psychological—and hence physiological—currency. With practice, this will become easier for you to do.

The Informed Power of Pictures

Most of us already know that a picture can speak a thousand words, but what do images actually do to your mind? Photos can affect the way we generate thoughts, feelings, and memories; and in just seconds (or less), they can trigger powerful and intense electrochemical changes, physically and mentally.

I recommend, for the most part, using color images as opposed to black and white. Color images usually (but not always) pack more of a punch, both electrically and chemically, throughout your body. They can change your brain-wave patterns (from high to low or vice versa) and alter your disposition from mellow to alert (or the other way around). A picture can help unify your whole body-mind-spirit connection and create a sense of flow throughout.

Moreover, a good energizing picture is certainly better for you (and longer lasting) than caffeine or pharmaceuticals, training your brain and mind to generate more of the natural energy you want when you want it—and without negative side effects. The reason for this is that, rather than simply activating your adrenal glands, the image reboots your mind-body with specific information, such as thoughts and emotions, which can be used to enhance a certain behavior.

Interestingly, you don't need to be actively looking at a picture to enjoy some of its benefits. In her book *Health: An Inside Job, an Outside Business*, Sonia Barrett quotes noted researcher and ophthalmologist Jacob Liberman as saying, "whether our eyes are open or closed, when we focus on something, our eyes respond exactly the same way."[1] In other words, it doesn't matter to your brain whether the image ramping up your psychological currency is right in front of you, in real time, or if you are picturing it in your mind.

TRY THIS!

Pick a photo you feel will give you the energy you need for your workday. As you look at the photo, ease your mind into its energy and feel the energy it is transferring to you. Take a few relaxed, deep breaths and feel the energy growing stronger. Then move your consciousness into the energy. Take a few slow, deep, and peaceful breaths; but don't exceed your comfort range. Feel the energy increasing in strength. Feel into it and cultivate it. Then take a deep, slow, and relaxed breath; and consciously ride the wave up to your forehead area and then to the crown of your head. Take a few more breaths and exhale each slowly.

If you don't feel anything (or much) from the image at first, it is okay, as this exercise can take practice. As you practice this skill, however, you will become better and faster at it. Also, once you feel the energy enough times to become familiar with it, you will discover that you don't need the image anymore. You will be able to call forth the energy by simply seeing the image with your mind.

When you feel you are ready, try performing this same activity with tri-level consciousness. First, feel the picture's energy within each space of your whole life being. Focus on the force and information the picture is delivering in each. Do this at a time and place when you can immediately make a few notations. Next, list (or think about) a few words to describe what kind of force you are feeling at each level—body, mind, spirit. Now, list (or think about) words to describe the force and information you are receiving from the photo and the force and information you are releasing from your body-mind-spirit.

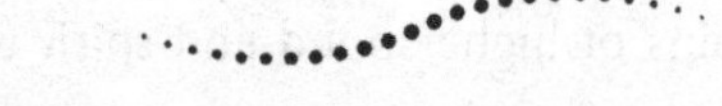

The Informed Power of Color

A certain color can quickly balance you or imbalance you. We know that your body radiates light. And this field of light that surrounds you energetically transmits, collects, processes, stores, and organizes your body's activity. This field of energy, which generally isn't easily visible without instruments, carries a full spectrum of color frequencies: red, orange, yellow, green, blue, indigo, and violet.

In holistic medicine, specific color frequencies are thought to influence your body and mind; and as a result, different colors can be used to regulate your being, as well as help with various psychological and physical problems. Color can increase or decrease your brain-wave activity, thereby moving you from high mental alertness to mellower states. It can help put you to sleep or drive you to anger. It can trigger the release of neurotransmitters that affect strength, focus, mental processing, and other functions.

Reds and yellows, for example, can stimulate your focus yet spark your anger, increase stress, and cause problems associated with overexcitability. Red can lift your physical and psychic (mental) energy, yellow your mental energy. These colors can affect both your *sympathetic nervous system*, which prepares you for quick-response action, and your *parasympathetic nervous system*, which activates a calming response.

According to holistic traditions, greens, blues, and browns, cool you down. Green can also, in some cases, eliminate a migraine.

Color, especially when combined with sound, can be used to target specific areas of your body at the cellular level, affecting the way cells communicate with each other, as well as the way your mind (at all levels, from physical to spiritual) orchestrates itself and then communicates with your body. As a result, color assists the transfer and transformation of energy from your other domains of higher mind and spirit to your biological body; each color can increase or decrease your energy. But the idea is to feel balanced and vibrant. For instance, bright red colors can stimulate and balance you if your physical and psychic energies are deficient. On the other hand, if they are excessive, they can have the opposite effect. In that case, if you are flooded with reds, incorporating or shifting to white rebalances you and returns you to your optimum. It's all about balance. Pay attention to what colors affect you in desirable ways and use them accordingly, to give you the energy you need. Experiment in situations of lesser importance.

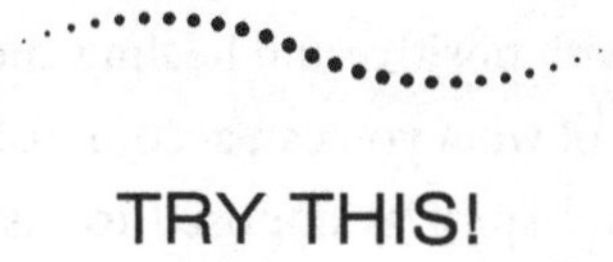

TRY THIS!

If possible, get up right now and have a loved one or close friend put a colorful sticker on your office key so that it is the first thing you see as you unlock your door. Feel into the positive energy it sends you with your whole-being awareness as you enter the office.

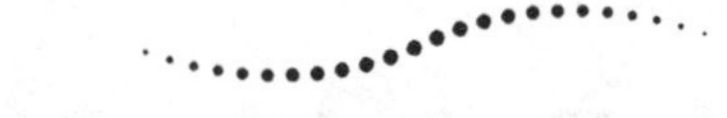

The Body-Mind-Spirit Energy Spectrum

As we have said, your *body-mind-spirit system* is your full living being. When this system is consciously unified and activated, you are able to cultivate psychological currency at each level and circulate it throughout your entire being. We have referred to this as tri-level consciousness. Becoming mindful in this way is at the core of this book. Your ability to feel into your full being, and input and output energy from any and all of its dimensions (as well as from and to anything around you), will make dramatic differences in the quality and amplification of the informed power you possess, cultivate, and share.

This kind of mindfulness can do more than just power you up for a given task. Such energy awareness helps you more fully understand your subtler energy capabilities as a living creature in this Universe. By understanding and using your subtler energies, you deepen not only how you see yourself (in terms of things that have happened to you in the past or will happen in the future) but also your meaning in life and in the lives of those around you. Choose to consider and regulate these subtle energies for use with future endeavors. In later chapters, you will see how the energetic changes you make now can influence events within your present, future, and even past with positive and healing energy.

Being more aware of what you can accomplish with your full energy spectrum of body-mind-spirit as opposed to just with that of any one dimension will also shape and deepen the way you see others, the things they do, and the way they feel. It will expand your understanding of interpersonal activities and their effects on you, and sharpen your decision making regarding them. We will do a lot more with these subtler energies in the coming pages. For the moment, let's start giving them attention and inviting them into your life.

Visualization

Visualization is another mechanism by which you can increase your psychological currency. Using a meditative mind-set, visualization employs a specific image or a series of images, like a movie, to help you "see" within your mind a subject or situation or task of your concern. It can incorporate as many of the senses as you like. I encourage a lot of sensory detail so you cultivate energy from each sense to give yourself the energy boost (informed power) you want for specific tasks.

Additionally, you can use visualizations to create new mental circuits to support and accomplish your goals, whatever they may be. For example, you might want to use visualization to sharpen your alertness when you need it, smooth your high-low-high swing pattern in tennis, or feel more animated when you arrive home after work. The possibilities are endless.

As was mentioned earlier in the chapter, it doesn't matter if what you are visualizing is happening in real time—right in front of you—or whether it is occurring in your mind. Through visualization, you can naturally and noninvasively activate specific brain networks (language, color, sound, motor); edit, short-circuit, or create new pathways for desirable behavioral responses; and create new connectivity and pathologies or strengthen old ones. Because of the brain's *plasticity*, you can literally remold your brain's operational system so that it is working in accordance with your desires.

Ultimately, when you practice this technique with tri-level consciousness, you get even more bang for your effort. Changes you've made in your body-mind-spirit connection will then activate similarly in real-time events when the situation for which you are training presents itself—like the act of taking the bus to work in the morning. For this to occur, you need to repeat the visualization often so that your mind gets the message that you want it to trigger the desired behaviors automatically. Essentially, you have created a new habit—only this one is entirely created in your mind, strategized and regulated by you.

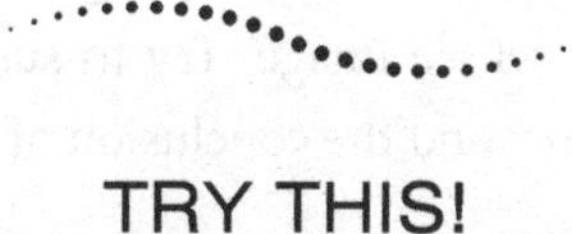

TRY THIS!

Using what we have discussed so far in this chapter, consider a variety of pictures you already have at your disposal that might energize you at the start of your day. Observe each image. Consider what it is about the images that gets your juices flowing. For example, you might get a boost from a memory associated with the subject, the colors, or the action pictured. Get as specific and plentiful as you can in identifying activators.

Now spend time visualizing each individual activator you've identified. Pick out the details that have a higher effect on you.

To amplify the effect, visualize the color red, yellow, or orange. Brighten and sharpen it as much as you can in your mind. Empty your mind of everything but that color, and just stay with it a bit. Flow with it. If you start thinking about other things, empty your mind again and fill it with your color.

Take a deep breath and inhale the whole color. Using your mind's eyes, see the color streaming throughout your body. Then, use your in-breath and internal vision again to stream the color throughout your intermediate (higher) mind, then your highest mind. Let the energy it brings awaken your whole being.

Once you are imagining it streaming through your highest mind, try to imagine it within all three levels of consciousness simultaneously. You may have a little difficulty at first, but with practice, you can get this—and it will be worth it.

Channel your chosen color and its energy downward, back through your intermediate mind, and into your physical body. Now, feel all three spaces energizing and sparkling simultaneously with each breath you take. Feel this color-filled energy surging throughout your whole being. Luxuriate within this. Feel the energy tingling at the crown of your head. Then slowly exhale the whole image. Try to sustain the unification of your body-mind-spirit beyond the conclusion of this exercises.

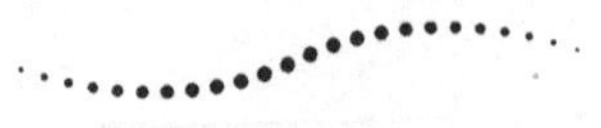

Music on Your Mind

Historically, throughout the world, music has been used as a way to tune the mind, heal the body, and heighten the spirit. Music is even viewed today as a way to connect with the Universe itself.

The reason it works is that the core elements of music—*rhythm*, *harmony*, *resonance*, *synchrony*, and *dissonance*—are the same components your brain uses to coordinate its own activities and behaviors. Music energetically permeates every part of the brain and can have a profound influence over its control systems, thus influencing your thoughts, actions, perceptions, emotions, memories, and neurochemistry. Using music, you can increase your energy levels before doing something requiring concentration or physical strength, or you can lower the frequency of your body's energy in preparation for sleep. It doesn't matter what type of music either; what does matter is that you like the piece. Also, the closer you listen to the song and its different parts, the more you can ramp up its effect on you. With practice, music can change how your higher brain operates and help you develop a whole new way of thinking about your world. As a result, you can use music's energetic elements to help you evolve into new perceptions and ways of doing things.

Music's Body-Mind-Spirit Connection

Your body-mind-spirit connection to music is amazing. Encoded deep into your memory are the subtle frequencies that ushered you into this physical life, carrying with them informed power from the higher realms of your mind-spirit and the Universe, embedding their rhythms and tempos into the first cells that made you *you.* As your first cells began to develop in the lush rhythms of your mother's heartbeat—the whooshing, low-frequency sounds pulsating from the placenta and umbilical cord—this beautiful and living symphony began *entraining* (two or more rhythms synchronizing into one) in your brain and organizing within your mind the primal soundtrack of your creation. These early musical influences stay with you for the rest of your life. Next to scent, music is the fastest way to reset your mind without drugs, and the effect is virtually instantaneous.

Additionally, from the perspective of mind-body medicine, specific musical frequencies can be used to help stream and transform particular energies from one area of the body-mind-spirit to another, as well as throughout your whole life being.

Beats per Minute

The term *BPM* in music refers to how many beats per minute occur in a particular song. For example, a song like "New York, New York," by Frank Sinatra, chimes in at a slow 27 BPM. On the other end of the scale, U2's "Pride (In the Name of Love)" comes in at a BPM of 106, and Elvis's "Jailhouse Rock" runs at a brisk 171. Then you get superfast tunes that can run over 200 BPM, such as "Boys of Summer" by The Ataris, which jets in at 201 BPM.

Using BPM to organize a personal playlist of songs you like is a fun and easy way to spike your alertness whenever necessary (the more you like the songs, the better they work). You can find BPM in many ways. The easiest is to simply do a Google search using the tags "BPM" and your song's title. Sometimes the Google search results will give you the BPM right in the listing. You can also find BPMs on iTunes.

Once you have the BPMs for the song(s) you want to use, I recommend arranging your playlist using songs from a lower to a higher BPM if your objective is to boost your general alertness. By doing this, you will increase your level of alertness with each song until you are optimally alert.

To identify the BPM I need for specific tasks, I break BPM into a spectrum of three ranges: alert (100–130), higher alert (135–155), and highest alert (160–175+). You can use this breakdown to make your playlists, and then load them on your iPod, cell phone, or other device so you can hit the play button upon need. Use your playlist often. The more frequently you listen to your playlist during a specific daily task, the more your mind gets the message that this is the level of alertness you want for this particular situation. Eventually, your mind will reprogram itself to hit this sweet spot for you all on its own, without needing the music. You'll feel positive results right away, but you'll feel more dramatic positive results within two or three weeks.

Why Music Works

One reason music is able to heighten your alertness is that you are in effect changing your brain-wave activity when you listen to it. Brain waves are electrical movements in the brain, and we measure these movements with an instrument called an electroencephalograph (EEG), which picks up the frequency of your brain waves through electrodes placed on your scalp. From the highest to the lowest, these frequencies are referred to as beta, alpha, theta, and delta waves.

Beta waves are active during your waking state—the one in which you feel most alert. In this state, your focus generally starts out alert and sharp, yet after you experience one concentrated thought after another, it generally dulls and you start to feel drained of energy.

Alpha waves are slower. They engender a feeling of calm alertness that is reflective and attentive. This is the state of mind often associated with meditation. Alpha waves support tri-level consciousness and receptivity to energy enhancing activities.

Theta waves are slower still. Referred to as "the dreamer's brain," theta waves are associated with a deep, relaxed state of mind in which you feel somewhere between wakefulness and sleep.

Delta waves are the lowest frequency. This is the state of mind in which deep, dreamless sleep occurs. It is the frequency associated with trances.

Generally, higher frequencies increase brain-wave activity toward greater alertness, and lower frequencies elicit more calm. The same has been found regarding the effects of BPM.

By changing certain frequencies and tempos in your music, you can move yourself through a spectrum of mental states that range from totally relaxed to completely alert, from low energy to high. Try listening to songs intended to increase your alertness for seven to ten minutes, and repeat if needed. Calming down takes a little longer—ten to twelve minutes—and can also be repeated if needed. You can pick the mind-set you want and sustain it. What's more, these changes have staying power. Ultimately, you can train your mind to automatically shift into these changes for specific daily situations.

Music's Emotional Connection

Emotional factors also influence how music affects you. These are generated from lyrics, messages, themes, and your ability to identify with something you can anticipate, such as the chorus or certain riffs. When using music to affect your energy, you want to be able to connect with something in the song that is sending you the right quality of alertness that you need for the situation you are in. The more you can make this connection, the greater the effect.

What this means is that while BPM is important, it isn't everything. There are times when your emotional connection to a song can trump BPM. For example, you might really like "Jailhouse Rock", but you may be able to achieve even higher states of psychic energy from the B-52s "Roam," which has a BPM of 135, because you associate the song with a fun-filled road trip you took with friends just out of high school. Furthermore, if a song's lyrics really excite you and bring you to the level of mental acuity you are looking for, that song can prove to be more effective than one of a higher BPM. So keep yourself open to this possibility when using music to reach a higher alertness.

Positive Physical Exercise

Exercise adds to both your psychological currency and physical energy. Everyone knows that regular exercise is good. In fact, it is a top-shelf morning activity to help boost your alertness. Anyone who exercises regularly knows that all you have to do is stop for a few days and you feel the difference. Even if you have health concerns, some form of appropriate exercise will increase your overall energy, help you fight back feelings of fatigue, and ultimately, help you live longer.

Physical exercise—walking, jogging, or playing your favorite sport—can deliver numerous benefits, including keeping your weight down, boosting your strength, and improving your cardiovascular system. Regular physical exercise is also a good way to help get your mind and body working together (in harmony) to allow you to step back as the day progresses and assess things with a positive objectivity—because you feel good and strong enough to push conflict at bay. This harmony allows you the opportunity to recharge, make adjustments in the way your day is unfolding, and then go at it again.

If you are looking for a substitute to energy drinks and processed energy foods, exercise is a good option. This is especially true when you make your exercise routine a priority, scheduling it on a regular basis and at the same time of day. Here's why:

When you schedule physical activity for the same time each day or week (mornings are best), your mind and body begin getting themselves "into the groove," so to speak, in advance. You can ramp up this process by using your tri-level connection to consciously remove energy blocks and more fully access your whole-being energy resources. This will help train your intermediate and higher mind to automatically remove any blocks and prepare your body for exercise. You can feel the difference this preparation makes.

For the best results, give yourself plenty of time to master this mindset during workouts. Lots of practice and repetition are important. As with any training program, this is because your mind recognizes your goals through repetition. For example, if you wake up at the same time each day, put on some running gear, and lace up your sneakers, your mind will get the message that you want to jog at that time and adjust itself to get things into place ahead of time. Your body chemistry will start changing to promote your alertness. Your body temperature will go up a little to help clear out toxins; and your heart rate, respiration, and the blood flow to your muscles will all increase to facilitate your run. Your warm-ups and cool-downs get programmed in as well, as does the alert and positive mind-set that you experience long into the rest of your day. Eventually, after a few outings, you'll find yourself waking up on schedule, without an alarm.

Loops You'll Love

You can increase the energy of any activity—in this case, those energies that boost your alertness—by anticipating its rewards. So, give good effort to keeping up your morning regimen. Put your focus on looking forward to and anticipating your healthy, feel-good activity. If you are jogging, anticipate your "runner's high" and how it will keep you glowing all day. Remember, anticipation creates reward loops and boosts the ultimate desired effects. Think of how much stronger and energized you will feel. Also think of how much happier and more social you are going to feel. Expect these perks, and love your activity!

These kinds of thoughts will spark your anticipation in preparation for and throughout your workout. It is one of the best ways to increase your endorphin and hormone production, which will help you achieve a high-definition mind that pays attention to details.

The more you engage in your exercise program, the more you will ingrain these feel-good expectations. In a short time, your anticipation—now informed with thoughts and feelings of alertness—will form an energy loop of anticipation, activity, reward; then more anticipation, more activity, and more reward. You are literally changing the way your mind and, hence, your brain will operate in the morning (or whenever you have scheduled your exercise time).

The more reward you induce and feel, the higher your levels of anticipation will spike. Many of the feel-good benefits you glean from your exercise will flow into other activities in which you engage throughout the day. These activities then create their own energy loops of anticipation followed by more reward. Every time you do this, every day you experience this way of living, you spike your craving for more positive experiences.

Conversely, you learn to reject negativity because it lowers the quality and strength of your energy, as well as your reward. This creates another good loop. Every time you block negativity from your life, you energetically feel rewarded. And you will anticipate this reward the next time negativity is knocking at your door—as long as you block it again, and so on. So, both you and your life pretty quickly start becoming more alert and more positive.

If you could see inside your mind when it is operating this way, you would see bright, sparkling, cascading, luscious, soothing, and simultaneously alerting energy. Close your eyes for a moment and enjoy such an image. Tell yourself you can—and will—live this way.

Exercise Fosters Better Nutrition

Another point to consider is how exercise affects your appetite. Daily morning and afternoon exercise helps you to make better nutritional choices. This is because you are feeling good and want to maintain that feeling. An old morning routine of coffee, television, protein bars, and negative emotional effects just won't look so appetizing anymore.

A morning exercise program triggers positivity, unblocks energy channels (depending on what form of activity you choose), and even curbs your appetite, making you feel good—mentally and physically—in ways you will relish and won't want to disrupt. By putting high-quality nutrients into your body, you are fueling yourself with similarly high-quality chemical energy, which you can use more effectively than the low-quality energy you might get from a protein bar. This will start another feedback loop for you as you begin to feel the psychological and physical rewards of good nutrition.

Too Much of a Good Thing

Once you engage your mind-body reward system, make yourself aware that rewards can also move you to overdo a good thing.

A track coach I know tells his class that running every single day is a good idea but not to the point of obsessing on it. Missing a day or more is totally fine. But some individuals become compulsive about their practice. There is a condition known as *exercise addiction*, and it is an easy pattern to get caught in.

Some people get so into their "routine" that, all of a sudden, there is no satiation point; and the activity hits a level well beyond negative returns. Ironically, energy input from excessive exercise reboots the body and mind to fatigue.

You know you are overdoing it when your exercise impairs normal functions, such as your ability to sleep or focus on tasks; or when you feel like you're going through withdrawal when you cut back on your activities. Some people find themselves trying to make up for missed routines when they skip a day or so. Feeling guilty, they may do two or three (or more) times as many reps or run much farther than usual. This kind of activity can send you a variety of messages to slow down, such as muscular, joint, and ligament distress, or anxiety and fatigue. Ignoring these signs can negate benefits and even lead to injury.

There is a time to push the limits of any performance to see if you can raise the bar, but this should be done with awareness and care. When your body and mind are ready, you can usually tell "this is the day." On the other hand, be on guard and avoid addictive patterns (as mentioned earlier). A good motto to follow: everything in moderation, including moderation.

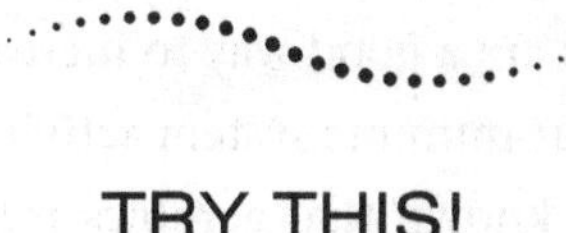

TRY THIS!

When your schedule won't permit exercise, there are still several things you can do to overcome sluggishness during the day. Catnaps are an easy way to restore energy, and they work fairly quickly. It's surprising, in fact, just how little of a catnap you need to feel energized again. Ten to fifteen minutes of consciously turning off your energy-draining activities will usually do the trick. However, it is important to note that too much downtime—say, over twenty minutes—can leave you groggy.

You can also try stepping away from your tasks and heading outdoors for a little while, especially on a bright, sunny day. Remember, light is energy. Just letting more natural light into your eyes reduces *melatonin* (the hormone making you feel groggy) and helps to pull you out of the blahs! I recommend taking brief walks outdoors for ten or fifteen minutes throughout the day.

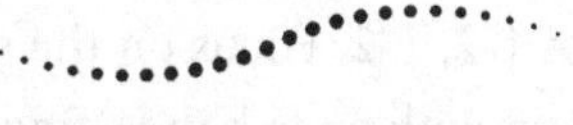

Aerobic Exercise

Aerobics are great for heightening the "voltage" on your alertness circuits. If you are looking for more of a lift with some staying power, this activity may be for you.

To be considered aerobic, your activity must be a *sustained exercise* (thirty to sixty minutes, three times a week) performed at a high enough intensity to increase and improve the amount of oxygen in your blood and strengthen the muscles, particularly your *large muscle groups.* Jogging, swimming, and rowing are typical aerobic activities.

Transforming the stored chemical energy from foods to heat and kinetic energy, aerobics are a good way to increase your alertness, gain stamina, strengthen your immune system activity, and ward off disease. Furthermore, it is well known that aerobics reduce the risks of many health conditions (such as strokes and certain types of cancer), boost HDL (good cholesterol) and lower LDL (bad cholesterol), and regulate blood pressure and blood sugar. Additionally, weight-bearing aerobic exercises, such as walking, reduce the risk of osteoporosis.

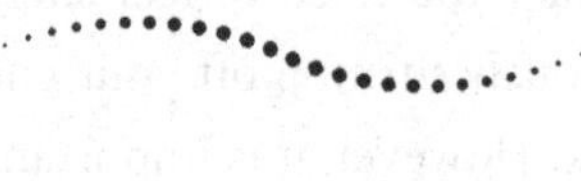

TRY THIS!

Stop reading for a moment and try out this very old kung-fu activity. (It is a wonderful energy- and focus-heightening exercise you can enjoy outdoors.) Get a bucket—or better yet, a water barrel—and fill it with cool, clean water. Don't get it so cold that the temp makes you uncomfortable, but try to keep it cool. Then, with clenched fists, smoothly—and lightly—punch with your left, then right hand into the water. Repeat many times to a rhythmic pattern of 1-2, 1-2. Focus on the sound and rhythm. You can also strike at the water with open hands, fingers together and fingertips aimed straight down. Try both, or whichever is most comfortable and energizing.

Try to empty all else from your mind but the sound of your fists hitting the water. Whenever you start thinking, just reel in your attention to the sounds of your hands punching into the water. Gradually speed up your strikes, and try to flow with the activity. This can be a refreshing way of simultaneously relaxing and energizing your mind in the morning or after work—especially during the warmer months.

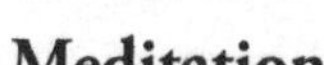

Meditation

Meditation is one way you can use mindfulness to regulate the way your mind is automatically activating various procedures, making them work for you more strategically, as well as deactivating ones that are disempowering. It is also the best way we have to cultivate more psychological currency, physical energy and spiritual energy, and ultimately achieve a greater level of alertness. Used properly, meditation will amplify the effects of all other methods of cultivating energy. It is an essential skill for achieving unity of body-mind-spirit and for accessing, transferring, and transforming energies throughout your whole being.

There are many types of meditation. The most popular type, however, is emptying your mind of thoughts, feelings, and voices; sitting with your eyes closed; and slowing and deepening your breathing in order to silence your mind. Whenever your attention wanders to a thought or an internal voice, reel it back in by focusing on the sound of your breathing. This is known as a concentration meditation. Your point of concentration can be the sound of your breathing or something else, such as an object, word, or color. Remember, these are all forms of energy, and they carry information and power you can use.

Another popular form of meditation involves widening your focus to take in the whole river of data coming at you. Here, you ready yourself as you did in the concentration meditation, yet rather than narrowing your focus to an object or the sound of your breathing, you are simply observing all of the information entering your field, trying not to judge, disturb, or attach to any of it as it flows through your mind. This is like watching thoughts, images, and feelings float across your mind as if they were leaves reflecting in a shimmering lake.

Both forms of meditation are effective, and many individuals practice them to relax or just get their mind off of things. The reason they work is because they slow you down, but they do not dilute alertness. In fact, your alertness should increase. Primarily, you are placing your thoughts and feelings in the background of your awareness and letting your pure, unthinking alertness flow into the foreground. You are energetically relaxed, yes, but you are also simultaneously increasing the crispness of your attention.

This combination of effects is why meditation is able to help you step back, take note of what's going on in a given moment, and find and activate the best operation or procedure to accomplish your imminent goal. It is also why meditation can help you edit or delete dysfunctional behaviors that increase conflict, stress, and dull the energy you need to sustain alertness.

Meditation detoxifies your body and increases the drive of clean, informed power through you, physically and mentally. With practice, it will leave you feeling tremendously alert and healthy—so much so that you will want to extend the effects of this mind-set.

Meditation Is an Energy-Building Mechanism

There is a reason why meditation practice is at the heart of enlightenment traditions, ancient medicines, and now, modern sciences and medicines. Meditation is more than a philosophical concept; it is the best energy-gaining and -enhancing mechanism we have as human beings.

By now, nearly everyone knows meditation is relaxing. But you can also use meditation to channel energy within your physical body, from one location to another—such as from your core to your limbs. Or you can channel energy from your mind into your body, enhancing your alertness or calm, or generating a broad range of other responses. Additionally, you can use meditation to transfer energy from your spiritual dimensions—from your highest mind downward, into your higher mind—and then issue it throughout your body and even outwardly, to affect others. So there are many more options than meditating solely to relax.

The more you practice emptying your conscious mind and turning off the messages coming from your subconscious mind, the more you will improve the overall quality and effectiveness of your meditation. This kind of repetition will send your mind and body the message that you want to create a new mental procedure capable of sailing you into this sweet mind-set in milliseconds and at selected times, especially if you practice your meditations before specific activities.

As your whole body-mind-spirit system enters a state of automatic flow, you begin to stream the right energy moment by moment, from each of its dimensions, directly to where you need it. In doing this, you are living the vivid, brilliant life that is our goal in *Body Intelligence*.

Your Original Energy Nature

We are all aware that virtue has a religious context. Although this is not the context in which I will be using the word in this discussion, I welcome anyone who wishes to think of virtue religiously.

Virtue, from a scientific perspective, is a subtle energy that pervades and harmonizes the entire Universe. It helps put a face on the Universe's spiritual energy as well as on yours.

Think about it: If you could husk your own energy to its purest nature, would you do it? Would you like to witness what is there? What would it be like? What would it feel like? What differences could this purest "you" make in your life—physical and otherwise? These are legitimate and important questions because opening up the pipeline to the subtle energy of Virtue will make significant and quick changes in your life and performance.

Indeed, your own purest nature and energy is the same as that of the Universe and that of the force and information from which you were born into this world. To describe this pure, original energy, the sages and masters of enlightenment have historically used words such as honesty, compassion, acceptance, peace, and unconditional love. These words have provided a way to understand the original characteristics of the Universe's energy and, in doing so, the informed power of its nature. Yet we know that the words, though energies themselves, are limited, as all words are. The feelings these words engender, however, are not. These feelings can help us experience, understand, and know this original energy further.

When you meditate on these words—and I highly encourage you to begin today if you have not already—try to feel into each of their specific energies. The closer you get to the informed power they hold, the closer you will be to your own original nature—who you really are.

The long ancestry of Asian medicines and philosophy has made human comprehension and the use of Universal energy a central focus in living well and meaningfully. From this view, human life, as all life, is not separate from the energy of the Universe. We are part of it. And it is intelligently (communicatively) part of us. Interestingly, there is currently significant agreement on this from the Western sciences as well.

To understand your own energy nature, you have to also consider the energy nature of all that surrounds you. Its purest nature is your purest nature—some traditions call this the soul. Feeling into this nature is feeling into the *ground zero* of you, your Self, the world around you and everything in it, and the informed core power of the Universe itself. This is the highest quality energy we know. When you feel it, you are energized, relaxed, safe, and happy.

As we have said, the words of Virtue—honesty, compassion, acceptance, peace, and unconditional love—are themselves energy (informed power). Theoretically, by attaching your mind energetically to these terms in meditations and visualizations—moreover, by feeling into them and living with them—you can remove energy blocks within you and reboot your entire being to its original default imprints. Successful rebooting will, of course, depend on several factors, including the quality of meditation practice to which you have evolved and your resonance with your original energy nature—Virtue.

However, because we live in and are part of this physical world, we cannot sustain this energy indefinitely. That is why individuals who use only the lower-level energy resources of physical life (such as medications) to calm down or energize, and even those who use subtler energies of meditations and visualizations as if these were medications for the physical body alone, achieve only temporary successes. In short, that kind of energy wears off like a pill; the problems just keep coming back. The reason for this is that the root cause and energy block exist beyond the physical body. Addressing the realms of body and physical mind only will not solve the issue; the energy quality is insufficient and the scope is incomplete.

Even though you probably won't be able to sustain your highest quality energy forever, you can still make long-lasting and even permanent changes in the way your mind and body function.

For the best results, you need to put in quality effort. I know that this is not always easy to do—for any of us. Yet in mindfully husking yourself down to your original energy to synchronizie your mind with the nature and goodness of the Universe, you can input the highest quality energy available to you. This is the energy that is who you are and have always been. When you choose to activate this energy, you effect a spectrum of changes in you, from electrical to biochemical, to the subtler energies, ranging from psychological to physical to spiritual. At the very least, this connectivity makes you feel healthy, whole, and good; and you shine through and through.

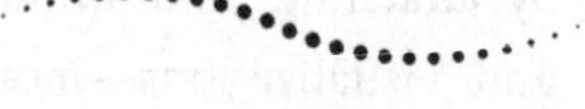

TRY THIS!

Take a moment right now to close your eyes and imagine yourself as you were when you were newly born. Simply imagine yourself comfortable and cozy, and warm all over. Use your mind to ease into the energy of that tiny being in your image. Don't touch the little person; just enter into its energy any way you imagine it. Settle into this energy and feel your way around in it. Empty your mind of any thoughts and just experience the energy that was you when you were first born: conscious and beautiful and alert. Now extend that energy outward, but try to remain sensitive to what you are feeling. Pick any one of these words: honesty, compassion, acceptance, peace, and unconditional love. Bring it to the center of your awareness and resist thinking about it; just feel into it. Feel how it positively affects your personal energy. Hold this energy for a few minutes or as long as you are comfortable. Then carry it in you and radiate it.

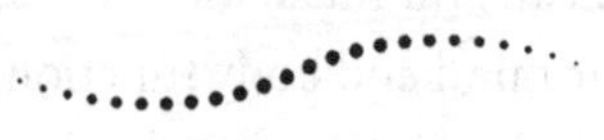

Living Virtuously

People who perceive themselves as acting virtuously gain energy physically—but there is more to it. Once you connect with the virtuous character of the Universe, you can refresh the energies of your body-mind-spirit. You transfer the subtle energy (of Virtue) downward from your spiritual level to the physical. Rebooting these spiritual templates opens up blocks that are making you operate dysfunctionally.

With these blocks gone, you automatically become more alert and feel better overall.

Beverly, a friend of mine, has recently experienced this phenomenon. She was diagnosed with PTSD and depression, and has felt weak and fatigued much of the time. However, she enjoys creative projects, such as the painting course she has enrolled in at a nearby college. She now thinks she'd like to pursue a degree in fine arts when she, as she put it, feels strong and alert again for longer durations.

A short time ago, Beverly joined an environmental group in her community. They go out on Saturday mornings, picking up litter alongside the highway. Besides cleaning up, her team collects returnable bottles. Surprisingly, the team has pooled together a considerable amount of money. They have currently extended their clean-up to include picking up litter at her college campus before anyone else gets to it, which has further increased the amount of money they take in. The entirety of the money then goes to a food pantry.

Beverly says she noticed herself becoming more vibrant as a result. She credits her environmental activities for making her feel good about herself again. This new sense of goodness and the robust energy she has been feeling are spreading into her week. As a result, her overall energy, especially the alertness she wants to sustain for her creative painting, has also increased. She has generated a positive energy loop with her creative activities, building on her newfound energy and increasing her vibrancy with her spike in creativity.

Additionally, feeling more energized, she now wants to help others do the same, so she attends a support group for individuals dealing with PTSD. She helps out by telling of her own experience. She provides guideposts and a lot of encouragement, using her own positive energy to motivate others. And this energy comes back to her, further empowering her and continuing the circle of good energy.

As Beverly's story demonstrates, once you change anything in any area of your full life-energy system for the better, you promote positive change throughout your whole being. But syncing and living into the energy with Virtue is essential; without this, any changes you achieve will be superficial.

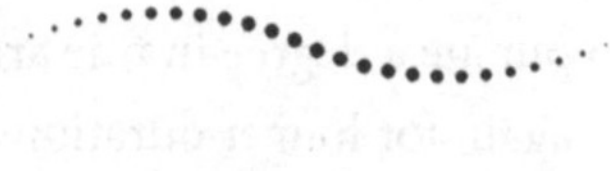

TRY THIS!

After you examine the chart below, take a few minutes to make your own chart. See what happens to your own energy when you synchronize your thoughts and actions with the high quality energy of Virtue. Notice the staying power of this positivity. Make this pattern part of your daily routine.

	BODY	MIND	SPIRIT
Acting trustworthy	More energy, healthier	Energized, balanced	Flowing, harmonized
Acting with compassion	More energy	Energized, balanced, happy	Flowing
Acting with acceptance	Healthier, alleviated muscle tightness, clearer head, more flexible, happier	Energized, balanced, higher self-esteem	Flowing, harmonized
Acting with unconditional love	Higher energy	Energized, balanced, happy	More satisfied, lively, flowing, harmonized and joyful; feel *I am good*
Acting with the thought: *Peace will be the outcome, no matter what*		Energized, balanced, happy	More satisfied, lively, flowing, harmonized and joyful; feel *I am good*

Energy Partners vs. Energy Vampires

There are people you encounter who literally boost your acuity as soon as you see them—or even anticipate seeing them. You get inspired by these individuals, learn from them, and often experience a surge in creativity after being around them. You intuitively know they are good for you.

Then there are those who suck the life right out of you. With some of these individuals, you are best connected only when in certain circumstances. For example, a certain friend can swing you out of a mood, but when you need to be really organized, that individual may not always make the best company. Other individuals, however, may be in a perpetual state of low, denser energy. If you know someone like this, that person may tend to cling to you, wanting to be around you more than you want to be around them. This is natural. It is because they enjoy the energy boost they get from you, yet you don't enjoy the energy drain you get from them.

The distinction between these two types of draining people is worth noting. A temporary pattern that has emerged because the person is dealing with a difficult issue does not mean that you need to cut that person out of your life. In contrast, people whose day-by-day pattern is draining your energy are probably caught in a lower energy that can be problematic for you.

However, it is possible that employment, social, or family reasons prevent you from isolating yourself from this individual. Or you may not be ready to disconnect. If one of these situations is true for you, then your job is to focus on staying in your zone when you are in shared spaces. Use your own energy skills to keep you in balance amidst any dysfunctional energy you are being invited into. You may need to cultivate a higher energy quality to do that. Unify your whole person: be aware, be virtuous, and be well. When you do, you can, in turn, energetically affect others around you to do the same, including those of lower energy. But whether you do affect them or not, you have cultivated more good energy for yourself that will sustain and strengthen you.

You can train your mind to do this, and with a little practice, you will eventually be able to do so anytime, without thinking. I suggest using any of the exercises within this book that seems appropriate to your situation. The power is ultimately yours.

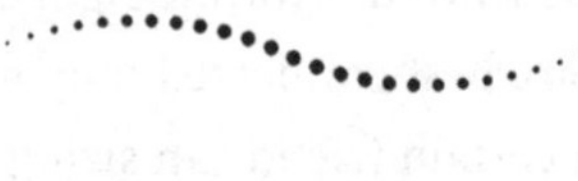

TRY THIS!

Close your eyes and relax for a moment. Feel into your own body's energy. Visualize it showering through you—bright, clean, high quality energy. Now visualize yourself as just this energy. Think of someone who heightens your psychic energy when they are around you. Take a deep breath and let that individual's energy flow through you. Let it revitalize and inform you. Feel into this energy you are cultivating. From a perspective of tri-level consciousness, see where this new energy download takes you. Feel it enhancing your own energy. Take a few more deep breaths. Channel the energy, using your breath to guide it to where you need it most within the body-mind-spirit matrix. When you feel your own energy heightening throughout, take a few deeper, refreshing breaths, and open your eyes.

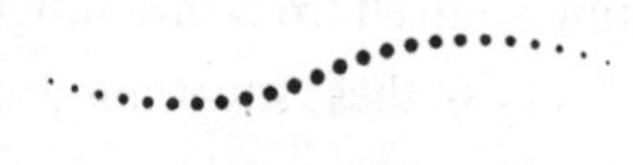

Swarm Energy

In nature, the collective motion, instantaneous decision making, and responses of swarm-animal communities seems so synchronized it looks scripted. One only has to look as far as a group of birds or bees or ants to see this informed power in operation.

In many ways, your mind can operate similarly. You are, at any given moment, under the influence of the various energies surrounding you and you can learn to use this connection to boost your alertness (as well as any of the other energy effects discussed in this book) and decrease its consumption.

Although it often feels like one unified current, you can widen your bandwidth and make yourself aware of the numerous energies entering your *personal energy field* (your whole being's energy) and influencing you. I call the combined flow of these strategic coordinated energies *swarm energy*. This flow can promote feelings and activities within and throughout all levels of body-mind-spirit.

In your everyday experiences, your mind pulls energy from a swarm of sources—anything in your external and internal environments—all at once (sound, temperature, scent, color, memory, feelings, words, other individuals, and so on). Yet you only need to focus on the particular source that you've moved to the front of your awareness. With swarm energy, the idea is to observe various things in your environments. As soon as you do this, you activate them. The more you feel into them and "listen" to their messages (effects on you), the more you can either let them in or inhibit them. Then you can start to anticipate looking at, listening to, and storing in memory those parts that have the most profound effects. And you can tap their energy when you need it in situationally specific moments.

You may find that some activating energies, if you stay with them too long, can be counterproductive to your goal of acquiring the energy boost you're looking for. Consider a painting on the wall in a café you may be working in. The painting arouses your alertness, yet keeping your attention on it too long sends you off on a reel of positive—though distracting—thoughts, feelings, and memories. Letting yourself feel into its initial energy boost briefly and then letting go of anything that follows can allow you to transfer this boost of alertness to your work, giving you greater energy, concentration, and flow.

To make this work, you need to avoid attaching to the distraction yet get close enough to feel its arousing effect. Stay centered on your goal; and once your energy has heightened, transfer the flowing mind-set.

Once you have activated several elements from your environment and Self (try using various senses), you can amplify the total mind-set. And you can do this by using all three levels of your consciousness. For example, you can use your breath to help you visualize the transfer of the positive, fresh energies you feel in your body up through your higher mind to your highest mind and then circulate them back to your body.

TRY THIS!

Let's energize various parts of your mind simultaneously to create swarm energy. Start by looking around your environment. Pick those elements that match the energy of your current task. Move the exact matches or most powerful energy match into the forefront of your awareness. Feel into its energy. Relax and regulate your breathing accordingly. Feel into all the energies at once, keeping the strongest influencer in the forefront. Stay with this for a few minutes. Clear your mind and flow with the energy.

You can use this activity at various points throughout the day to sharpen your alertness. Additionally, you will discover that some environments will have a lot more energy sources to promote your activities than others. Note these and match them with specific activities.

Exercises and Practices

1. Use BPM (and music's emotional factors) to make a playlist of your favorite songs that you feel can give you the alertness you will need on the way to work tomorrow. Put your playlist on your iPod or cell phone and use it.

2. Hydrate yourself before breakfast tomorrow. Then step outside for a brisk walk or short jog. Or if you like, try out some Eastern movement like chi kung, tai chi, or yoga. Combine your exercise with sound or scent. Peppermint works nicely to stimulate you.

3. Engage in an early morning aerobic activity of your choice. Then follow that with a relaxing, energy-building activity like tai chi or yoga for ten to twenty minutes.

4. Try this energy booster and de-stressor in a standing or seated position. Relax and regulate your breathing. Hold your right hand out, palm down, about a foot in front of your chin. Now trace the infinity figure with it, starting from the right. Do this a few times and then engage your left hand, starting just an inch or two behind your right hand. With both hands engaged, keep this going for a few minutes.

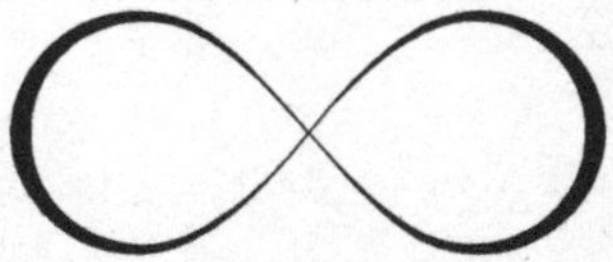

5. Take breaks outside today, especially if it is sunny. Any natural setting will work. Incorporate scent. Experiment with different settings and scents.

6. Locate a bright environment (with lots of natural light) where you can go for lunch. Treat yourself to that place today.

7. Meditate and feel into your most remembered, perfect, alert energy. For you, this may be a charged athletic or musical event, or any significant moment (particularly new experiences) in your personal or family life. Ingrain this image and energy in your memory by recalling it several times during the day. Then use it to charge your alertness in specific situations.

8. Look at a word or a color or a picture. Visualize it as pure energy. You may see, for example, that its energy looks like a line—jagged, crooked, or straight—or perhaps like a soft light green, or nearly translucent like rain, or black and opaque. Now look at something in your environment that energizes your alertness such as a painting, a building, a tree, a garden, or even something like a doorknob, lamppost, or electrical outlet. See it as electrical current. Give it a color, pattern, and linear movement. Feel into it. Use your breath to draw it into yourself. Feel this energy. Let it heighten your alertness. Commit this energy to memory.

9. Make a list of people and words that energize you. Bring them to the forefront of your awareness whenever you want to heighten your alertness at various times during the day.

5

USING ENERGY TO REVERSE STRESS

Energy and persistence conquer all things.

—Benjamin Franklin

While optimal amounts of tension and worry can be motivating in preparing yourself for an activity, enhancing the drive to hit your goal, too much tension will result in stress.

Stress is what happens when you experience relentless tension. The danger is that as your stress escalates, you can experience numerous negative effects, including demoralization, loss of appetite, and depression. Other manifestations of stress include pain, nausea, fatigue, difficulty breathing, and amnesia.

Once tension becomes stress, you lose your sense of flow and joy, and perform below your optimal level. In fact, your higher level energies of mind and spirit constrict or block. As a result, stress leaves you to perform at the most superficial level, draining your overall available energy.

This pattern is difficult to overcome, restricting your growth as a whole person and even causing serious illness.

Be Aware of Quick Changes

All kinds of rapid change in your life can stress you out. For example, maybe you or someone you know suddenly experiences illness, the loss of a loved one, or new employment. The stress might even be due to a good cause, such as graduating from college or forming a new romantic relationship. How you react to such changes will determine whether you will be affected negatively or not.

Again, becoming aware is a good first step in dealing with stressful energy. You can then support it with calming energy (force and information) and a change in your perceptive lens.

Extinguishing the influence of the major cause(s) of your stress is one possible path for dealing with it. But if that's not in your interests or if that's just not a realistic possibility, then adapting to it until you can extinguish it is another way to deal with it.

Each of these paths require certain energy. Also, this energy will be specific to you. In order to relieve the stress you are experiencing, you may need to first calm yourself down. But then, let's say that your stress is the result of gridlock; you may also need to charge up more physical and mental energies to get unstuck and overcome it. This energy should send the particular messages you need to hear in the moment to give you the force and guidance you need.

The Right Kind of Energy Support

Max, a former high school teacher, recently took an early retirement. He was only fifty-five. But his job had been stressing him out for years, and he was determined to do something about it.

He didn't want to stop work completely, however; he was was looking to work at something different and less stressful for the second half of his life. He'd planned for several years before his actual date of retirement. So when he hit the magic age of fifty-five, he was ready to fly.

Max now wanted to work as a consultant. During his years teaching, he was very good at writing grants for himself and for the elementary school where he worked. He loved accruing money for what he considered worthy projects. This was one of those things he did that made him feel good about himself and brought into the light of day a piece of who he really is.

More than once during his career as an elementary school teacher, Max had experienced family as well as community heartbreak over a child contracting incurable disease. Now Max, in his retirement, decided that he wanted to turn his grant-writing talents toward amassing monies to help in medical pediatric research.

He took a position at a nearby hospital, where he was given an office and staff to help him seek funding for research in pediatrics. This was exactly what Max was looking for. So it was "surprising" for Max (his word) when, one day, he woke up to the realization that he was stressed beyond belief—worse than when he was working forty-hour weeks teaching. He didn't know where all the tension was coming from. To him, it didn't make sense. He was even having trouble getting a good night's sleep.

You hear similar things from individuals who have gotten themselves out of a detrimental relationship and into a new and healthy one—how can this be stressful? It's supposed to be what you want, right?

Max started drinking a little more wine with dinner to handle the stress. That staved it off briefly, but then his insomnia got worse, and he was groggier the next day. He wondered why he was stressing—after all, he was only spending around fifteen hours a week at the new office. The rest of his time involved non-work-related activities.

When Max started his new job, everything seemed great. He was creating his own hours. Once he'd get the kids off to school, he and his wife spent their days off together, usually taking short day trips to fun places. For Max, spending time with his partner is an energy gain, as it should be for any of us in a good relationship.

The days Max spent with his wife out in the fresh air, bright natural light, and in fun places had a soothing and replenishing effect. They made his workdays feel lighter; they were an energy gain as well as a stress neutralizer. He had, in fact, slept a little less those nights, yet had more energy and slept better. We all need to balance stress by shutting off our energy-draining pipeline and turning on the energy-gaining pipeline.

Then things changed for Max. The changes were slow yet steady, and with them, came a stream of tension.

Max's wife started getting called into work more frequently, cutting down on their recreational time together. With the sudden surplus of home time, Max decided to do extra work from home. As his energy declined, he faced other issues that were new to him—mostly idiosyncrasies of his job. The tensions mounted and weren't going away. Most important, Max wasn't gathering any new supporting energy to soothe them. This created an imbalance that left him feeling wired—worse than when he was working full-time. Max would now start his days with a shortage of energy, which was not being refreshed. Tasks that used to feel like a piece of cake now seemed strained.

You cannot let yourself get into this kind of tailspin if you want to stay physically and mentally healthy, as well as energized, flowing, and happy. You need to make yourself aware and then make necessary adjustments.

To prevent this kind of nonrestorative cycle, give priority to the ways in which you decompress pressures and recharge your full being energy. This may mean finding ways to take breaks, to get away from the stressful environment, or to create opportunities to blow off steam and play, both at the workplace and after. Somewhere in your mix of fixes, you should include meditation and reflection, not only to increase awareness but also to put you in touch with your whole life being, recharging you with clean, fresh energy.

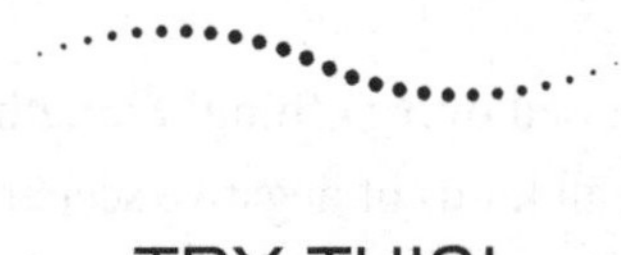

TRY THIS!

Take time right now to think over your agenda for tomorrow. Identify one or two predictable situations that will use up larger amounts of your energy. Then plan a bit of a recharging activity before or after your energy drains (but preferably both). If you can't arrange this schedule, find ways to take little breaks during the energy-consuming activity. Get to a different environment and do something restorative. Read something creative or spiritual and of high interest and pleasure for you. Maybe you like to listen to audiobooks. Try meditating or listening to a piece of music that sends you the right messages to restore your energy, and finish your day happy. Or do something creative, like sketch a natural scene. Go slow—take the time to enjoy what you are doing. Notice these are all activities that fuel your spirit. Let these activities and your other production-driven mind-set relax and restore you.

Before you go back to your work, focus on your highest-level mind (spirit) and breathe deeply, slowly, and calmly. Now envision the energy you have cultivated within your highest mind, stream it downward into your higher mind, and then into your physical body. Feel the energy enter your body from the crown of your head and stream it throughout your entire body, then circulate it back up and loop it down again several times. Feel this high-quality, natural energy flowing through all the levels of your being. Luxuriate in the moment. Let it unify and restore you. Remember the feeling.

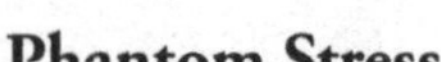

Phantom Stress

Do you ever get all stressed over nothing? Sometimes your imagination gets you stressing over all kinds of negative scenarios that could happen to you but never will. *Phantom stress* is the result of both electrical and chemical activity in your mind and body. Individuals with phobias experience this feeling and get caught in it.

Say you are afraid of snakes. Then you've probably experienced walking along and suddenly thinking you see a snake right in your path. Your reaction is virtually instantaneous. Within a millisecond, you are in the throes of your fight-or-flight response, streaming an electrochemical storm inside you.

It doesn't have to be an insect or animal phobia, however. Similar responses can occur just walking through a crowded shopping mall and suddenly seeing (or thinking you see) someone you really don't want to bump into. These and similar kinds of stressful reactions are often inflated and inaccurate, but they all turn on your energy-draining pipeline to full blast and cause a lot of unnecessary stress.

What's more, when we are thinking this way, odds are we're probably wrong in our assessment—wrong around 99 percent of the time! In fact, when you are already fearful of something, you tend to see it even when it is not there. Nature has wired us with this fuzzy circuitry for a reason.

Maybe when you were young, a one-foot-long, yellow-and-black snake almost bit you (or did). So you file the object as "dangerous snake" in an emotional memory that is very fuzzy. To see how this memory system works (and how it doesn't), imagine making a photocopy of a picture on an old analog photocopying machine. Then imagine taking a photocopy of "the copy" and repeating that process a few times over. After a while, all distinguishing features in the photo start to disappear. In the end, you may only see some dark shading and a few lines here and there. If you were doing this with a page of print, for instance, an *O* would decay into what may look like a *C* after making a few copies of copies; you wouldn't be able to distinguish between an *L* and an *I*. This is how your emotional memory records things—fuzzy.

Although it may seem counterintuitive, this is where nature's genius reveals itself. Consider what would happen if evolution had given us high definition fight-or-flight memory. Say you could memorize feared objects with such high definition and specificity that you could recall the most intricate of details with absolute clarity. If this were the case and you'd previously been bitten by a one-foot-long, yellow-and-black snake, you would deposit those specific details in your memory. Then if, sometime later, you encountered a seven-foot-long, brown-colored snake with diamond shapes on its back, your highly accurate memory would give you a free pass, assuming that dangerous snakes are all one foot long and yellow and black. Your fight-or-flight response would not kick in, and you wouldn't see and feel any threat—at least not yet. However, you may be looking straight into the eyes of a diamondback rattlesnake that's about to attack you.

By keeping a fuzzy image of your feared object in memory, nature activates your fight-or-flight response whenever anything even remotely resembling the object of your fear presents itself, making your assessment and response often inaccurate, yet protecting you in the one situation when they are accurate.

Fear-based memory is so powerful that you can be roaming around an environment full of positive and pleasing objects with only a single fearful object, and your mind will locate that fearful object faster than any of the others. This is why a frowning (or disgusted-looking) face in a crowd of smiling people will stand out even though there are many more happy faces.

What this essentially means is that nice things will distract you from things you don't find fearful or stressful, but they won't interrupt you when it comes to things you do fear. But this pattern isn't good when you are trying to bust stress in your life. This is because each positive element, even though it may be irrelevant to the task you are trying to concentrate on, is relevant to you and your whole energy cultivation.

Scientifically there is reason for the expression "stop and smell the roses." In fact, any positive sensory elements within your immediate environment are energetically useful when it comes to taking your attention off the stress you may be experiencing. This allows you to refuel while slowing down energy consumption. It may also offer energetic information to enable you to further deal with your task more fluidly. By ignoring the positive energies in your environment, you may be turning yourself off to both the information you need and to the calming force of those neutralizing energies. Opening yourself up and seeing and feeling into these energies can refresh and rebalance you.

Western Energy Balance

There are various meanings for the term *balance* with regard to energy. From a Western scientific perspective, balance refers to an optimum state of mind between calm and alert.

You may ask, what's optimal? Your mind is balanced when you are operating in a mind-set that is in a middle ground between an activated, focused state and a calm, relaxed one. To enter into this state, your brain has to be able to make adjustments. Staying in this middle ground keeps your physical and mental activity flowing. If you were to be any calmer, for example, you would be too mellow for the specific situation you're in, and if you were any more alert, you'd be too wired. Adjustments are made per and amidst tasks or goals to keep you in your balanced (optimum) mind-set.

You may, for example, need a certain amount of energy to prepare a meal from scratch and more relaxed energy to enjoy the meal you've prepared; so, somewhere along the line, you need to adjust or shift energy. In another instance, you may require a certain quality of robust and organizational energy to get yourself out the door and into your car in the morning, yet a mix of calm but alert energy as you drive out into traffic and head to work. Remember, it takes longer to calm down when using relaxing techniques that it does to become alert.

From the Western perspective, you can adjust and manage changes in balance by working with your brain's electrochemical components—e.g., brain-wave and neurochemical activity—which we have been discussing and will continue to discuss in coming pages. When you cannot adjust, you feel imbalanced, and this imbalance brings on tension. When that tension persists, you experience stress. Imbalance blocks necessary force and information, which then snowballs to create additional stress. So feeling imbalances as they occur is a good thing because it provides you with the opportunity to stop stress in its tracks. The danger in allowing imbalance to continue is that it can sweep you away into dysfunction or even begin to feel normal to you, leading you down paths that are harmful without your awareness.

Holistic Energy Balance

In mind-body medicine and many holistic arts, we enjoy the idea of balance as an optimally performing mind-set. We add the Universal Principle of yin-yang to the Western perspective as an essential element for fully understanding the concept of balance. This is because the concept of yin-yang provides a very clear picture of energy as it exists in all things, from biggest to smallest; the force and information that comprises it; and its continuous momentum.

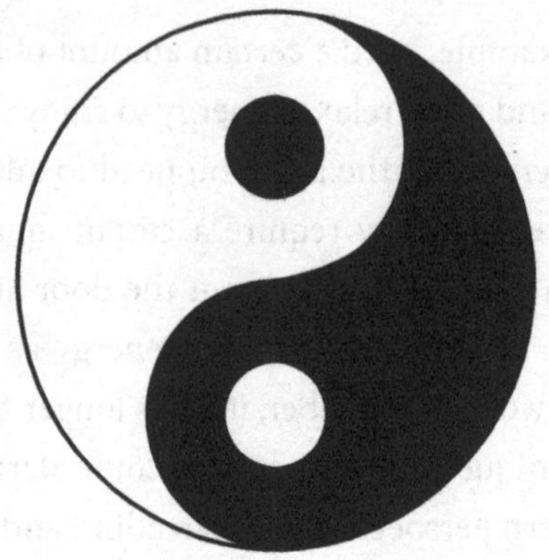

The circle of the yin-yang symbol represents the energetically cooperative nature of all things. In holistic medicine, we consider this energetic cooperation *Universal Law*: the concept applies to all things in the Universe—ourselves and all we do included. The dark color in the symbol refers to yin, the female universal energy within all things, from the tiniest particle to the Universe itself. The light color refers to yang, the universal male energy, also within all things. Here, the terms male and female refer to specific energies, not gender. Notice that within the symbol's dark coloration, there is a dot of light; and in the light coloration, there is a dot of dark. Conceptually, this refers to the universal need for (and balance of) both yin and yang everywhere we can see and beyond. You can't have one (yin or yang) without the other. You need both (yin-yang) for balance and harmony.

Balance is an essential and serious concept in holistic medicine and in Asian traditions. The word China translates to "middle," "center," or "middle kingdom." As with many concepts based in these traditions, there are layers of meaning below the superficial, and many benefits to cultivate and grow. In a similar manner, martial arts practitioners study a *form* or *posture* only to learn four years later, when they think they have mastered it, that there is another, more advanced form—with deeper concept and benefit—then another and another. In the West, we can become frustrated with this idea—when a student earns a degree, many believe this means they are done with their education. I have personally heard many individuals saying things similar to, "Okay, that's it—done with that. Now I'm ready for something else."

In Eastern traditions like karate, earning a black belt indicates that you have mastered only the basics of your art. That is why students are told the story that in the most traditional martial arts, there was only one belt: the white belt. As the story goes, the white belt, after much experience (naturally soiling and tattering), turned black, indicating the wearer had achieved a certain level of mastery; but as her experience continued, the student's black belt would continue tattering until it turned white again. And the circle continues: to black then white, over and over and over. Traditionally, the karate student sees the dojo as just a smaller representation of what happens in life.

This kind of balance—this continuous journey of yin-yang, of body-mind-spirit, of informed power—is what you learn to pursue; it is not a trophy. Through cultivation and growth, you transform your personal energy from low to high, and learn to sustain this high-quality energy, health, spiritedness, and joy throughout your life and beyond. This pursuit is, in fact, connected to our ultimate purpose in life. For this reason, I want to get more specific about yin-yang.

The Nature of Yin-and-Yang Energy

First, notice the term *yin-yang* is hyphenated. This is done purposefully. It indicates that you do not want one without the other, and that you need both for balance. You can be a person, for example, who is soft (yin) yet unyielding (yang), a person of backbone (yang) yet not hardened (yin). Harmony balances opposites, and balancing opposites energetically results in harmony. Just as day turns to night, and night to day, and just as the seasons change, so it is with the body, mind, and spirit. There is no conflict, stress, or stagnation when you are balanced. Your energy and life flow.

You can consider the nature of yin as the Universe's reproductive energy. Yang's nature is, on the other hand, productive. Yang refers to issues of exterior and heat, whereas yin refers to interior and cold. Yin's physical and psychological problems have to do with cold, deficiency, and low energy; whereas yang has to do with excessive energy—e.g., type A fiery personality and overexcitability.

The principle of yin-yang can also help you to see more clearly and better regulate your personal energy patterns—how they are functioning and affecting you. For example, an individual's high-energy appearance may be because he is yin deficient, which makes him seem to have jumpy, excessive energy. You see this often when someone is burnt out, has stayed up all night, is full of coffee, and is scrambling in frustration. Their yang (productive energy drain) is straining, overheating, and draining, not really excessive. Look at the symbol again. As yang energy wanes, it naturally wants to shift to yin—as yin will "cool it off" and facilitate its restoration. When someone is burnt out, it may be that their yin (reproductive, cooling, restorative, energy-gaining pipeline) is and has been deficient, and as such, can't refuel the person's energy output. The yang energy is, however, what you are left to see on the surface. At the extreme of either yin or yang, you naturally and energetically want to enter the other.

For balance: yang-excessive needs energy to "bleed off" the overabundance of fire-heat in the individual, whereas yin-deficient requires cultivation of the person's yin energy. These are not interchangeable. If someone is yin-deficient hyperactive, you won't get good results by taking a jog, which will make the person's yang energy strain even more.

If, on the other hand, the person is yang-excessive, the jog will achieve the balancing result you want, staving off some (or all) of the excessive energy. Chemical treatments, whether pharmaceutical or in the form of caffeine or energy drinks, can be problematic for the yang-excessive person in the same way an exercise like jogging can contribute to further imbalance for the yin-deficient person. Also, even when chemical treatments are appropriately used, they provide only temporary solutions, and sometimes compound problems with undesirable side effects.

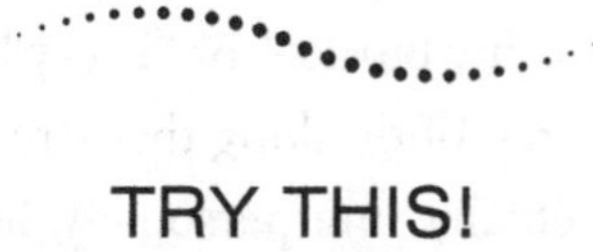

TRY THIS!

For one whole day, complement the actions of your environment, whether they are generated by a person, place, or circumstance. Don't barge into a place. If someone speaks, listen. Relax when the traffic light turns red. When you are the next person in line at the store, don't hand the cashier your money until he or she is ready and shifts into the "receive" mode. Use your passive mode to build energy, then filter it down to your active mode to spend it. Be both soft and powerful. Be strong and fluid.

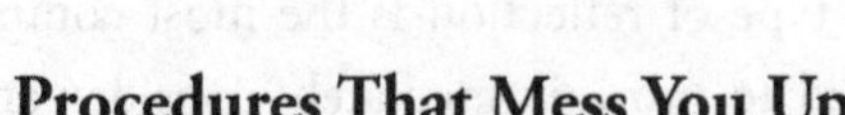

Procedures That Mess You Up

Sometimes stress and loss of calm originate from behavioral templates that mess you up. Like the teacher in chapter 2, you may be speaking to someone who seems to be staring out the window. That person may actually be thinking about what you are saying, but their seeming lack of interest in your words fires your frustration circuits and streams adrenaline into your bloodstream. Next thing you know, you are derailed, saying or thinking something you may regret. The problem in dealing with this stress is that we aren't always aware of its connection to our habits. Remember, these templates fire in a virtual instant—in milliseconds. Therefore, their relationship to how we are feeling or how things are working out for us may go unnoticed.

What we do notice is the stress that *dysfunctional behavioral templates* cause in our lives. Sometimes, we get so used to operating under the influence of these processes that our actions and emotions, including all of our stressors, feel normal to us. I'm sure you have heard individuals using the phrase, "This is my burden" or "Every life has its tribulations." It's easy to fall into the trap of thinking that stress is part of the turf we tread upon—environmentally, interpersonally, intellectually, physically, emotionally, and spiritually. If, on the other hand, it turns out that the turf itself is stressing you out, you need to make some adjustments. You can start by looking both internally and externally.

What You Can Do for Relief

Check to see if your stressors are the result of dysfunctional templates. If so, begin removing them. You can do this by practicing reflection, looking back with an open mind into endeavors that fall short of your goals or that don't work out, and even those that do work out yet you still wish to improve. This type of reflection is the most common. Sometimes, however, you need to more immediately consider and regulate your thoughts, feelings, and actions. For this, you can also practice reflection on the fly.

But you can also practice reflection on the fly. Although it is a little more difficult, this kind of reflection can be done within an activity, making adjustments to improve your performance as you go along. Most of the time, though, dysfunctional templates kick in so fast, you feel there is no stopping them. And though it may seem impossible, you can, with preliminary practice, stop them and the stress they generate. A good place to start practicing is by taking some relaxed, mindful time later in your day to look over the situations that brought you stress. By tracing the dysfunctional behaviors associated with your stress, you can be on alert for them when they pop up in other real-time scenarios in the future.

The key to success is in knowing the peripheral energetic signs of stress. This knowledge gives you a cue when a specific template is about to bring you trouble and helps you replace it with one that will achieve better results.

It isn't easy to do this at first, but you can learn with just a little practice. Because dysfunctional templates trigger so quickly, it's hard to become aware of them midflight. However, through mindful reflection later in your day, you determine what state your mind and body were in just moments before you engaged in the behavior that stressed you out. The behavior may have been a thought, feeling, or action (remember, these are all energetic events). This information makes you conscious of early links in the chain of events and information that streamed through your mind and led up to the actual behavior. Once you are able to identify the links (symptoms), you can train yourself to stop their progression before the stress-causing behavior occurs.

Ultimately, you want to replace a dysfunctional template with a healthier one. Then you must train your mind to use it as your mind's default setting. By replacing the faulty template with your new functional one and using it repeatedly, you will short-circuit the early link, create a new brain circuit with the healthier template, and establish a whole different—in this case, stress-free—outcome.

At that point, your new behavior will automatically engage every time afterward when you are in a similar situation. You might be thinking, "That sounds like a lot of work." But it really isn't, because you are going to do it little by little.

Mindful reflection is a great way to identify your stress buttons and knock them out one by one. Day by day, week by week, your energy gain, positivity, and overall performance will begin to soar.

Jocelyn, a former workshop participant of mine, told me that when she practiced this type of reflection, she discovered that her fear of being reprimanded for lateness, which has been with her for as long as she can remember, is a major link in a chain of events that leads to daily stress. Her stress then manifests into arguments with coworkers and loved ones.

By stepping back from doing anything more than observing within these moments, she was able to finally notice some of the peripheral symptoms of her stress: her face flushes, her voice rises in pitch, her body movements stiffen, and her desire to use bawdy language increases. Additionally, incidents that made her tardy in the past start flying through her mind. Making herself aware of these early cues has helped her intercede and shift into a better mind-set.

TRY THIS!

For one day, make yourself aware of the situations that are stressing you most. Step back, take a look at one of them, and observe what exactly is going on. Don't analyze or put labels on anything. Just see, hear, and feel into the situation.

Later, when you can calmly reflect, use your mind to revisit the situation. Let the details and your involvement in the situation unravel step by step. Put your attention on what was happening right before the stress triggered—when you hit the almost-stressed point. Ask yourself: *What was happening to me physically, inside my body? What was I thinking and feeling? If my reaction was seen by others, how might they have seen it? What behav-*

iors could I have engaged that may have changed the course of the oncoming stress? See yourself in the situation again but with these new behaviors.

All of this information will help you identify the moment before the faulty procedure kicks in. And with practice, you can begin to identify it earlier and replace it with a happier one.

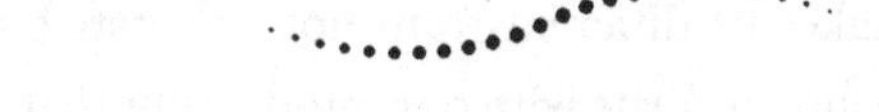

Visualization Is the Human Difference

One thing that makes humans different from all other creatures is our ability to create a total fiction in our mind and use that scene to parallel what we want to happen in real life, seeing what works and what doesn't (in terms of our goals) and then making a decision. This uniquely human quality is based on our brain's attention network, which relies on information we have stored in memory, external information that is available to us, and how we gather this information together to find solutions. Visualization makes it possible to identify a dysfunctional mental template and replace it with a better one—one that will enable us to avoid stress.

For example, say you put a rat in a box with a green light and a lever in the front of the box (in psychology, we call this a Skinner Box, named after the behavioral psychologist B. F. Skinner). If the rat pushes the lever when the green light goes on, it gets fed Purina Rat Chow (there really is such a thing). You can train the rat to do this.

Now, let's put me into the same box, only let's reward me with one-hundred-dollar bills instead of the Purina Rat Chow. I push the lever one thousand times and make $100,000. The rat matches me and is now looking well fed. Then one day, you tell me that you are going to put a red light in the front of the box. You inform me that when the red light goes off, a lethal electric shock will be delivered through the lever. When I see the red light go on, no matter whether I want the one-hundred-dollar bill or not, I will visualize in my mind what will happen to me if I touch the lever, and I will choose to stay away from it. The rat, in contrast, having been rewarded with rat chow one thousand times, will see the red light go on and go for it.

But don't feel bad for the rats. They do well for themselves, living conditioned lives. We humans, on the other hand, like choice.

One thing that makes us different from not only rats but also from other animals is this ability to create with our mind events that haven't happened. We, unlike other creatures, can tune in to imagined scenarios and have feelings and thoughts about them; consider a variety of probabilities; and then, all things considered, "think about" and decide how we want our experiences to go. Combining these tools with mindful reflection helps you connect what happens to you as the result of your procedures, desires, and urges; and helps you make more conscious choices. It allows you to feel in control, keep from stressing out, and gain more high quality energy.

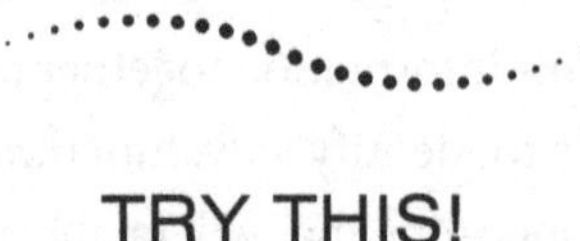

TRY THIS!

During a quiet, relaxed moment at the end of your day, close your eyes and reflect on how things went for you. Think of more significant events first, as they are easiest to consider. See if, at any point, you might have handled or responded to things differently.

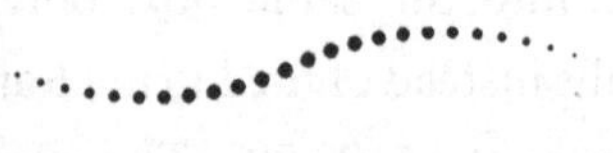

Understanding the Self

Earlier, we discussed that your mind is flooded with eleven million bits of data per second and that, at maximum attention, you can handle around forty bits. Nonetheless, if you do the math, you will see that forty bits of information is a huge number when stretching it out over an average lifetime. Even half that sum—because who is maximally attentive all day long?—is still a lot of data from which we have to make choices. I have come to the conclusion that these moments of awareness and choice are, in a way, sacred moments. They comprise, in fact, the unique canvas of our life in this world. To choose authentically, we have to choose from the core of who we are, which includes an accurate understanding of Self—as you view yourself in past experiences, as you exist now, and as you see yourself in the future. When you live this way, you feel balanced, stressless, and as though you are living full of purpose. So much of the stress and unhappiness individuals experience in life comes from losing connection with Self. But what is this part of us that we call Self?

Self can be defined as your representations of your own personality—the various parts of your character: behavior, temperament, and so on. Self can also refer to the "I" Self, or pure awareness—to the execution of your consciousness. Some world traditions consider this realm of pure conscious awareness your original Self, or original life being or spirit—your soul.

From the perspective of holistic medicine, Self refers to the perfect, conscious, energetic unification (integration) of your whole living being of body-mind-spirit. And this is where the concepts of energy, center, and balance come into play.

The Energy of Bliss

"Follow your bliss"[1] was an anthem made popular by the mythologist Joseph Campbell. Mind-body medicine also addresses this idea of bliss but from a scientific perspective. This view allows us to take the notion of bliss a few steps further in understanding why it is an important aspect of living a stress-free life.

Bliss is related to the idea of Self because when you are mindfully operating within your Self, fully aware of the informed power of your highest mind vibrantly and brilliantly flowing through all three levels of your consciousness, what you experience—what you feel—is bliss. This feeling is perhaps as opposite of stress as one could ever get. Bliss is what it feels like to be operating in sync with your original nature. When you operate from this whole-being vantage point, rather than draining energy, you gain energy. Rather than living in conflict with who you are, you live without stress, authentically—flowing your full living being with others and the things you do.

However, following your bliss does not mean, from a mind-body medicine perspective, that we should all go out and become hedonists in any realm, be it the body, mind, or spirit. Some people allow themselves (their attention) to attach to things. When this happens, you lose the wider view as well as your ability to regulate your focus, because it is attached to energy other than your own genuine consciousness flowing with it. Attached, your mind and life start working like a guided missile, with your attention or mindfulness following the "thing" you've attached it to instead of you, your Self. This pattern is true, loud, and clear in all addictions, and it removes the possibility of conscious self-regulation and flow. Furthermore, it uses up the energy you need to create your life. But this pattern goes beyond addiction and includes anything you attach to, such as owning a certain vehicle, attaining certain employment, and so on. This generates a huge stress point: a conflict between your original nature—your deepest Self—and the way you are living and feeling day by day. This conflict also blocks access to your higher energies, and furthers the strain and drain of your lower energy resources.

To follow your bliss, you have to put your attention inward. Go back to the original clean, uncontaminated, stress-free slate of your original Self. One way to achieve this is by practicing mindful breathing. Focus on your in-breath as though you are tracing it with your index finger, streaming your awareness through to your human mind, into your higher mind, and into your highest (spiritual) mind, which is where your true and first nature exists—your bliss. By mindfully exhaling, you are further able to touch this brilliant informed power as it cascades through all realms of your whole living being.

As you witness and journey within this space more and more, you will discover that the place you have been journeying to is what the great masters of enlightenment have referred to as the heart of your very being. When you mindfully exhale from this vantage point, you can extend your awareness beyond yourself without perimeters. And then you will uncover the big discovery that this place—the heart of you—is also the seat (the heart) of the Universe. Your heart is its heart and its heart is yours, simultaneously. On that day, which will come for you with practice and cultivation, you will consciously experience the center (the source) of all energy. You will be one and the same.

Within this view, when you are centered within your full being of tri-level consciousness, you are in and experiencing your bliss; from there, you will get the right force and the right message—from there, you cannot go wrong. If you trust in anything, trust in the blissful intelligence of the Universe. Trust in the direction in which it is naturally flowing you. The more hectic and stressed life becomes, the more important it is to feel into and flow with this energy. Make yourself aware, witness, energize, be, and then do. Feel your stress vaporize.

Virtue

Entering the energy of Virtue and simultaneously letting it circulate throughout your full life being is an additional (and necessary) way to achieve, amplify, and balance calmness. Just as the energy of Virtue works as an exciter, it also calms you. This is because you are consciously filling yourself and operating with the natures (Virtues) of Universal energy—its driving force and information. We have identified these natures as honesty, compassion, acceptance, tolerance, peace, and love.

Living in sync with this energy reboots you to your being's original energy state, activating your energy-gaining mechanisms, and thereby eliminating stress and even sicknesses. As this high quality energy—its force and information—streams from your spirit through your mind and into your body, it strengthens the right aspects of your physical and mental nature, and creates new circuits (procedures and processes) to guide you toward better health, satisfaction, longevity, and happiness.

Changing Your Energy Ratio

Once you change your energy ratio to a point of higher quality and balanced energy by using any of the techniques discussed thus far, your next job is to sustain it.

As you become more and more de-stressed and energized, check in on your improvement often. You will feel, for example, as if you are going from 50 percent stress to 30, 20, 10 percent, and lower. What you want is to feel that your positive energy (calm and alerting) is going up at the same time from 50 percent to 60, 70, 80, 90 percent, or even better.

You want to lock into this higher energy zone so that you don't just feel better momentarily, going back to your old stressed-out, energy-draining lifestyle. Unfortunately, many people are prone to getting themselves over the hump and then going back to where they started—or worse: going further downward so that they are operating below a positive, balanced energy level of 50 percent. I hear about this digressive pattern often. Some people, for instance, say they have a morning routine to get themselves started in a positive direction (like jogging or walking); but then, as soon as they get into their car and head into traffic to get to work, they lose the healthy mind-set they just cultivated. And it's a dysfunctioning mind-set they take into work with them. Or they cultivate energy for long periods of time, operating at an 80 percent energy level, and then digress.

When we use up our positive energy, rigidity settles in, resulting in shallow satisfaction or no satisfaction—sometimes even irritation and depression, and little to no joy. If allowed to continue long enough, a negative energy loop results, and various physical or psychological sicknesses can follow.

What you want to do instead: protect the bump in positivity and balance you've gained, and keep it going. When you feel yourself tipping off balance, one way or another, correct the imbalance with more alerting or relaxing energy, whichever you need—so that the scale doesn't tip so far in one way. And if it does, attend to it before it becomes an ingrained daily pattern. Make the sustainable, healthy energy pattern your reward. Then make that into an energy loop—your new feel-good, rewarding pattern. With practice, your mind will start to go there on its own. Your flowing mind will create a flowing life.

Aligning Your Activities with Your Goals

Moving forward in the things you do while having a feeling that you are living with purpose also prevents stress, as this perspective turns on your higher-quality energy pipeline. When you feel that your daily activities are helping you achieve your deeper goals in living, you feel the higher-quality balanced energy streaming through you—from your highest mind downward, to this physical realm. You ward off and lose stressors. You feel a connection between your dreams, your actions and thinking, and where you are heading in life.

For this connection to be authentic, perceptions weigh in; you can't really fake it. You have to get past a conditioned mind-set—what everyone else wants for you—and instead, listen to and explore your Self. Otherwise, your higher quality energy is blocked. You know it is blocked when you cannot get past the superficial level of the physical (lower) realm. Symptoms of a blockage can take many negative forms, including conflict, lack of satisfaction with life, and attraction to self-gratification rather than cultivation. In Asian medicine, these all link up into what is known as karmic energy, so that, at some point, the force and information of one's life then determines like action and the consequences that go along with them.

Experiencing purposeful living can be likened to going through life as if you are in a boat effortlessly traveling in smooth, gleaming water; knowing you are headed toward something that is deeply part of you and your ultimate goals. There is reason behind your movement and momentum and you feel it in each passing mile. When your life is operating thusly, you don't relentlessly stress out. In fact, you gain positive energy within its flow. You continuously set your own energy bar higher and enjoy the journey of reaching it.

To create this state of living, you have to first put in the time to understand your Self and what you really need to be doing, as well as where you need to be heading. Chasing things that are unnecessary depletes your energy and leads to stress, blocking (cutting off) the downward flow of your higher energy of spirit and mind. Furthermore, if you aren't truly focused on what you need to do, purposeful living becomes more like happenstance and can then add to your stressors. Thus, mindful reflection that helps you see your true Self and evolution is necessary in all that you do.

TRY THIS!

Ask yourself if the universal Virtues of honesty, compassion, acceptance, tolerance, peace, and love are present at all three levels of your consciousness: body, mind, spirit. Think about how and where they are present, as well as where they may not be sufficiently present. Which of your endeavors and desires in the physical realm are, in truth, necessary—real needs—and which are not? Remember, chasing things that are unnecessary depletes your energy and leads to stress. Reflect on ways you can begin to incorporate Virtue into your life today. Visualize how good you will feel sharing this energy in your daily activities. Feel into and activate this energy often throughout your day.

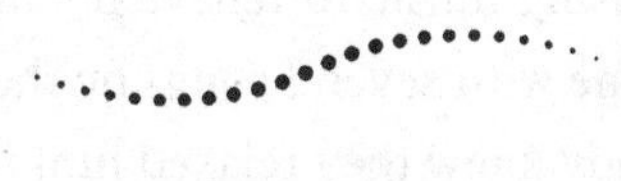

Music

As we discussed earlier, music can be used to influence your body's electrical and chemical energies to induce alertness. But it can also be used to heighten calm and pleasure. Relaxing songs trigger the neurochemical *dopamine*, which is the body's natural, feel-good hormone. Dopamine, which is associated with feelings of euphoria, is able to reduce levels of stress (and even chronic pain) by increasing the feeling of pleasure in response to certain thoughts or actions. The calming capability of dopamine is so powerful it would require a license to prescribe it. If you were to view a scan of your brain during a cascade of dopamine brought on by music, the similarity to brain images of someone using cocaine would be uncanny.

Ever hear someone humming or whistling during tense moments? Singing, chanting, whistling, and even humming can bring on the release of this self-produced brain drug. Once you associate the euphoric feeling with the tune, you are doubly rewarded with more dopamine. You'll feel this calming pleasure throughout your entire body and mind. You just have to like the tune, and as we have said, the more you like it, the better it will work.

Medicinal Musical Rhythms

Music can change your rhythms from those associated with high stress (high beta) to those associated with low stress (alpha and theta) in a millisecond. So you can (if you enjoy them) use songs like "Every Breath You Take" by The Police or "First Spring Day" by Mia Jang to unclutter your mind. Listening to Mozart works well for many individuals too.

One such individual—Jack—struggled with insomnia for several years. Then he tried using music to relieve his nighttime anxieties. He loaded up his cell phone with several songs he thought might calm him down because he already knew they relaxed him in other scenarios. Not all of the songs worked for this particular goal, but the one that finally did the trick for him was "Reflection Eternal" by Nujabes. He would lay back in bed, close his eyes, and play his calming song for about twelve minutes each night (or a little more if necessary), before turning off the lights and going to sleep. As the days went by, he started feeling better and better. After about three months, he started using the song randomly. "I don't need it all the time," he said. "It's like my mind starts playing it all on its own. Next thing you know, I'm out."

When using music to lower your stress, be sure to choose songs with fewer than one hundred beats per minute (BPM). The lower the song's BPM, the better. For example, Norah Jones's "You Turn Me On" has 59 BPM. Instrumental pieces and those with lyrics will both work, but if you choose songs with lyrics, make sure they're sending the right message.

In addition, you should strive for songs that you already know have a calming effect on you, or songs that had a calming effect on your mother while you were still in the womb. Songs from childhood that carry a safe and warm coziness, such as those you sang with your parents before bed, also have a calming effect. But remember: no matter what you choose, you have to like the song—and the more you like it, the better it will work.

Other Calming Practices in Conjunction with Music

Try adding visualizations to your music sessions. Create a comforting interpersonal image or environmental image in your mind as you listen; or make a mental movie.

Use color. Visualize the color green as you listen, or imagine a natural environmental setting with luscious greens. Then view it as though you were looking through a green lens. Relax, slow, and deepen your breathing; breathe the entire image in. Feel its calming energy.

Sometimes playing white noise for a while before your playlist will help shut off your mind (you can purchase recordings of white noise online). You can also shift out of a detrimental mind-set by using a slideshow of a time and place where your mind felt perfectly free, happy, and relaxed. Then put on your insomnia-soothing playlist.

Using recordings of nature's soothing sounds works well too—wind or rain, a campfire, a waterfall, or ocean waves are all favorites. Plan ahead with these by making your playlist ahead of time, so it will be available whenever you need it.

Swarm Energy to Calm

Knowing how to use your mind to find the calm within yourself and within other things allows you to call upon this energy for support and balance whenever you need it.

Furthermore, just as you harnessed swarm energy to help you reach higher levels of alertness, you can do the same to help you relax and calm down. The formula is the same: begin by paying attention and sensitizing yourself to those elements in your external and internal environments that have a calming effect on you. Feeling into their energy, you invite their calming force and information into you. And you can do this with anything in your environment; you don't have to limit yourself to landscapes or sounds or colors and so on.

You can focus on anything at all, such as a word, phrase, or a tool—anything. Practice feeling the myriad of these energies and practice often, so that you ingrain them in your memory. Try to feel the various energies under the influence of different frames of mind—e.g., when you are elated, sad, jumpy, burnt out—to discover which of these energy sources works best with each of your states of mind and in specific situations.

Consider keeping a record of the things that work best for you. A good way to do this is to collect photos and images of the energy sources. You can then store these on an electronic device, such as a cell phone or iPod, so that you can conveniently retrieve and practice orchestrating your swarm of calming energy whenever necessary.

Introverts and Extroverts

On one level, it is popular to understand extroverts as garnering more of the energy they need from outward interaction and introverts from within. From the perspective of holistic medicine, however, this approach can be hit or miss. It ultimately depends on the circumstances, which can vary widely.

If an extrovert requires a superficial lift, then yes, being around people can work—even if it is chit-chatty socializing. The bit of stress relief you gather may be enough to hold you over until you get to a better source—and may be your best alternative at the moment. Yet too much of this surface interaction can take you off course and further drain your energy, giving you less thinking power with which to resolve the conflicts causing you stress. Eventually, you have to flow back to purposeful activity; straying away for too long creates its own kind of energy drain or stress.

More important, if you are an extrovert who has cultivated a high energy level of both higher and spiritual mind, then you will not be sufficiently satisfied with a peripheral or superficial (lower) energy interaction. Finding yourself losing more energy than you are receiving, you will feel greater stress rather than relief. Everything cannot be in depth all the time. So the answer for you may be to participate in chitchat while gauging how much energy you put into the interaction. For example, it can be good to deliver some energy to the others and receive some in return. However, although you may be increasing your lower energy to an extent, you may not be increasing your higher quality energy much.

Part of energy training is expanding your energy resources. As such, the extrovert may benefit more from trying some artistic, athletic, or other mentally stimulating activity that also involves a social component. This way, you are enjoying the pleasure of a social environment while doubling up on your energy gain with more energy-building activity. This will enable you to bleed off the negative/stressful energy, fill with positive energy, and build your creative energy supply.

An introvert, however, may not fare as well when participating in chitchatty social situations to decrease stress. Instead, he may require some time alone. If this is you, you may glean more from creative activity, daydreaming, singing, chanting, dance, scientific and spiritual discovery—energizing experiences in solitude. It is better to stay clear of negatively charged individuals when you are stressed or to limit your time with them. A better solution: spend time around those you know well who share in dreams and deeper, meaningful talk. Their positive energy will balance your own. Try to do the same for them when they need balance.

As either an introvert or an extrovert, make more time to get away for a breather during your day. Incorporate your right-brain activities during these relaxed moments. Don't use time off to ruminate. Focus on opting for peaceful resolutions in times of conflict, and think about how good you will feel coming out on the high road.

Empty Mind

There are times when you need to eliminate stress on the spot. *Empty mind* is a coveted mind-set conveyed to us by the grand masters of martial arts and Eastern philosophy. This concept and technique is also utilized by other holistic arts, mind-body medicine, and traditional Asian medicines. It is intended to bypass stress, attachments, and other negative feelings—even on the fly. As a result, your full consciousness can open freely and get involved in the transfer and transformation of high quality energy to match your pursuits.

By employing the empty-mind technique, you train your mind to guide you in the pursuit of authentic needs; this, in turn, will energize you with the force, information, and reward loops you need, moment by moment.

To help me understand the idea of empty mind, a martial-arts master once told me a story about a famous Japanese swordsman, Miyamoto Musashi. According to Musashi, your attention must always be in a state of flow. If it stops anywhere, for any reason, the flow is interrupted, and it is this interruption that deteriorates your awareness. For the swordsman, deterioration of awareness means death. When a swordsman stands against an opponent, she is not to think about her enemy, herself, or the movement of swords. She must think of nothing, and let what is in the unconscious surface and take over.

Beginner's Mind

Beginner's mind is a concept from Zen Buddhism (though it also used in holistic medicine and arts) that says if you want to learn anything well, you must attain the simple focus of an infant, whose mind is empty and fresh. This mind-set has no preconceived ideas; it sees things as they are and is free from the procedures of experience—and therefore, open to all possibilities.

Beginner's mind may sound a lot like empty mind (*Mushin*, in Japanese), but it is a different tool. An infant's mind is like a sack of clear, vibrant consciousness—without any derivatives. Pure, alert, and flowing, this is the consciousness with which we are born. Empty mind is a tool in our energy toolbox that we can use repeatedly to wash our slate clean of faulty perceptions and procedures, and drop into beginner's mind when necessary.

TRY THIS!

Take a moment to meditate. Slow down and deepen your breathing. As you breathe in, say in your mind, "It feels good to breathe." When you release your breath say, "I am fully here." Then empty your mind of all thoughts, emotions, and desires; and take the elevator down to your *lower dan tien*. This major location of energy is located a few inches above your navel and, interestingly, is your body's center point of gravity. Relax; breathe slowly and evenly; feel the enjoyment of your breathing. Then extend your awareness (consciousness) outward through your higher mind and into your spiritual mind. Keep an objective (silent witnessing) mind-set. Feel clean, positive energy. Let this enter and surge within you. Observe everything that enters your awareness objectively, as if it is reflecting on the shiny surface of a clear, sparkling lake. Pass no judgment. Eliminate all else that enters your mind. Just watch and go deeper into the energy within this field.

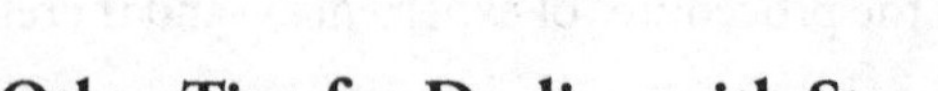

Other Tips for Dealing with Stress

When stressors start building, tell yourself that the overwhelming odds are that things are not as bad as you imagine. This anxious, fear-based feeling is usually inaccurate (remember the snake on page 94). Slowly breathe in and out a few times. By changing your perspective, you will feel yourself naturally soften. Give yourself permission to have a lighter perception of the stressing issue.

Humor works well to ward off stressors, whether your stress is internally or externally generated, or whether it is spontaneous or planned via reflection. Try reading a comical text or creating a humorous playlist from your favorite comedy YouTube videos. You can also create a humorous musical playlist or an album of your favorite personal photos, or combine the two. One thing I find works well is to have another family member create a humorous slideshow of you, using a funny soundtrack and putting it on your iPod or cell phone. My daughter created one of these for another member of our family and mailed it to him in the middle of an extra-stressful week, and it worked wonders.

Use mindfulness to prepare for potential stressors in advance. For example, if you will be introducing a new contract at a business meeting and you know there will be objection, think it through beforehand. Prepare a working plan to deflect the objections. Perhaps you can address areas of predictable conflict and eliminate them before they become problematic.

By pairing various body-mind-spirit concepts and techniques such as the Universal Principle of yin-yang and the energies of movement in order to reach a balanced calmness, you can train your mind and body to stay calm and alert and flowing. By using various methods, you will also give their effects more staying power. Being able to sustain this mind-set will allow you to transform stress into tranquility. For some people, it can mean being able to transform a hell on earth into paradise.

Exercises and Practices

1. Try this stress-busting acupoint meditation. Sit on the front edge of a chair, keeping your back and head straight and well postured—as though there were a string attached to the crown of your head, pulling you upward. Keep your feet flat on the floor. Place your hands on your lap, with your left hand palm up on top of your right hand (also palm up) if you are male, opposite hands if female. Be relaxed all over. Close your eyes, and breathe abdominally and slowly. Put your focus on the *Bubbling Well* (center-of-the-foot acupuncture point) of your left foot if you are male, right foot if you are female. Sit in this position for five to ten minutes, and smile as you focus on the acupoint. As your mind focuses on this acupuncture point, you will eliminate stressors. Smiling during this technique in any meditation will activate various (positive) supporting electrochemical responses throughout the body. Also, you can often find great relief using this technique when you wake up at night and think you may have trouble getting back to sleep.

2. Before going for your morning energy drink, try feeling into a calming energy first. Use any of the calming techniques in this chapter—from music to visuals. These activities will help keep your brain waves in an alpha range and away from the higher beta waves associated with anxiety and stress. They will also trigger the biochemical reactions that will help ward off tensions, and generate and sustain a feel-good, flowing mind-set. Go through a few morning routines slower than usual, taking your time so that you are

not expending so much energy. In fact, this will help you conserve energy. Then try your energizing drink or other energy resources. You may have to work this routine a few times in order to break away from automatic expectations and habits. You may also find this process only works on certain mornings. Note those times, and use this method for them.

3. Use a five-star system to see how effective different things (images, sounds, narratives) are in reducing your stress.

4. Use a blood-pressure machine to track your blood pressure and heart rate with various stress-reversing activities, so that you can see which activities work, how fast, and under what conditions, as some may work better in specific instances than others.

5. Actively do nothing for a whole day. Empty your mind, and intake calming energies all day.

6

USING ENERGY TO REVERSE HARMFUL MOODS

The image is more than an idea. It is a vortex or cluster of fused ideas and is endowed with energy.

—Ezra Pound

Emotions are an example of informed power. They are natural and basic to all. Some emotions affect your body-mind-spirit like a magic elixir, bringing you quality energy with which to get things done—and right—and making you feel on top of your game. Other times, your feelings can be downright detrimental. You may find yourself wondering just what you have to do to get out of their influence. It's like spinning your wheels in mud. You think, *Why can't I just put away my feelings and get on with things?*

But emotions are an essential part of who you are and how you perform. So you can't just pitch them aside. At some point, you have to confront and deal with them in a way that is energetically advantageous for you and anyone else concerned. Knowing a little bit about how emotions work on your mind and body will help you do this.

Negative Moods

It's easy to fall into a negative mood. And this shower of high-speed electrical and biochemical activity can throw a lot of weight in how your life goes. A coworker says something critical and you feel hurt. A family member neglects to acknowledge something you have achieved and yet compliments another family member for something they've done, and you feel slighted. You feel a coworker should agree with you about a certain financial issue but he doesn't, so you get irritated. These and other negative feelings can trigger negative moods so fast they are often virtually automatic. What's more, they can have their roots in old habits (templates) that are stored in your memory and fire at gut level, so to speak, before you ever get a chance to rationally think about what you are feeling and whether you want that specific influence. All under your radar, these old templates trigger unreasonable thoughts, actions—more unreasonable feelings.

By seeing your feelings as energy, force, and information capable of fueling your everyday endeavors and development (or not), you can begin to better regulate and benefit from them. You can also learn to use your positive energy sources to reverse a mood that has become detrimental, enhancing those that are functional. With a little practice, you can soon start to disengage damaging moods within yourself—and even with your partner—within seconds, and get back the clarity and fluidity you want.

The Informed Power of Feelings

We have known for many years that emotions affect the operation of your body and mind. Because this influence extends over your whole life being of body-mind-spirit—its health and interactions—it is important to identify downward moods when you get into them.

The animal kingdom provides many examples of the extraordinary influence of feelings on health and behavior, and has been the subject of a wide range of studies regarding this issue. For example, in 1992, D. C. Lay wrote an amazing account in the *Journal of Animal Science* that cited the raw power of emotions in the animal kingdom.[1] Using cattle who were not accustomed to handling, Dr. Lay zeroed in on what happened when these cattle were placed in a restraining device for branding. What he found was that the fear-stress induced by restraint raised the cattle's cortisol (stress hormone) levels almost as high as the levels brought about by the hot-iron branding itself.

According to doctors Alan Rozanski, James A. Blumenthal, and Jay Kaplan, extensive evidence from animal studies (especially the cynomolgus monkey) reveals that chronic psychosocial stress can lead to a host of severe physical maladies, ranging from reproductive issues to heart disease.[2]

What's more, research shows there have been numerous stress-related animal deaths, including nearly 50,000–80,000 worker bees who were so stressed out by their queen bee's death that they "left en masse to die."[3] Elephants in captivity have been reported to die much younger than their counterparts in the wild. In an article in *The Guardian*, researchers warned that lack of exercise and stress were killing elephants. "Scientists also blamed high stress levels, which the animals suffer most after being transferred between zoos and being separated from their mothers."[4]

Similarly, veterinarians I have spoken with on this subject noticed that exposure to fear-stress also takes a toll on the immune system, compromising its overall ability to fight off infection. But the physical damage suffered from emotional responses is not just a veterinary thing. Humans suffer from their feelings too—sometimes even fatally.

Back in 1986, there was a story of a forty-four-year-old woman who was admitted to Massachusetts General Hospital.[5] Although she had felt fine all day, in the afternoon, she developed extreme, crushing pain in her chest and radiating through her left arm. This is a classic sign of a heart attack, but strangely, she didn't suffer from coronary heart disease. There was no life-threatening clot in the arteries surrounding the heart. Describing the unusual case in *The New England Journal of Medicine*, Drs. Thomas Ryan and John Fallon suggested the apparent damage to the heart muscle was emotional rather than physiological, stemming from an incident earlier that day, when she had been informed that her seventeen-year-old son had committed suicide.[6]

I remember hearing of a similar incident that occurred when I was a boy in the early seventies and a young man suddenly died without warnings of previous illness. His mother, upon hearing the news of her son's death, died herself, almost immediately. That evening, rather than having one casket as was previously scheduled, the funeral home had two side by side—mother and son. Stories of living beings dying from a broken heart abound.

The effects of trauma, particularly PTSD, have been taking their toll on US troops returning from deployment in Iraq and Afghanistan. CNN reported on November 14, 2013, that, according to Department of Veteran's Affairs calculations, "Every day, twenty-two veterans take their own lives. That's a suicide every sixty-five minutes." CNN further stated in that "a survey by the Iraq and Afghanistan veterans of America showed that 30 percent of service members have considered taking their own life, and 45 percent said they know an Iraq or Afghanistan veteran who has attempted suicide."[7]

From the perspective of mind-body medicine, excess negative emotions and even positive emotions can be harmful not only to the body but also to the mind and spirit. We further know that a deficit of positive emotions can also be damaging. For these reasons, I suggest that you step back and become aware of what you are feeling, especially before and after important daily situations. Make balancing the connections between how you feel (emotionally), how you think and act, how healthy you are, and how you can become even healthier (and as a result, live longer) part of your daily reflections.

The Five Emotions

We in mind-body medicine believe there are five universal emotions that affect our internal organs as well as our mind. These emotions are joy, worry, grief, fear, and anger. While it is normal and healthy for us to feel these emotions, our response to them determines whether their effect on us is detrimental or positive.

Joy affects the heart, keeping it strong and warm. It also maintains balance in the small intestines, decreasing tension and increasing the flow of blood and energy. A balanced amount of joy, influenced by the ebb and flow of certain hormones in the blood, will optimize your focus, memory, and self-esteem, and help keep your body-mind-spirit flowing. This activity is especially important as you age because these hormones will start to register lower on your dipstick over time. When balanced, joy streams relaxed and calm yet vibrant and stimulating energy through you. The tricky part is learning how to maintain joy in balance, as this energy can easily become excessive and dysfunctional.

In excess, joy can lead to hyperexcited behavior, resulting in rocky thinking, poor decision making, and potentially harmful activity. Balancing involves making yourself aware and having some calming energy techniques at hand, to help you level off when needed. In contrast, too little joy or a sudden drop from higher joy can spiral into downward moods and depression, fatigue and insomnia, as well as other physical and psychological problems. You can realize your ultimate and balanced joy when you put your mind in a state of quiet observation (during meditation) at your highest energy level—that of your spiritual mind. When you practice this kind of meditation, your whole mind becomes clearer and happier, and your body stronger and healthier.

Worry affects the spleen and stomach. In small amounts, worry can be a good thing. For example, if you didn't worry a little about your health, you might eat sugar- and fat-laden foods for every meal. A little worry can also induce sharper focus, comprehension, and execution of information. Excessive worry, on the other hand, causes depression and stagnation of your physical and psychic energy. This can result in a failure of the spleen and stomach to transporting nutrients to the rest of the body. Common symptoms include rapid pulse, depression, anxiety, weakness of the limbs, poor sleep, and loss of memory. As we discussed in the previous chapter, once worry becomes relentless, it can be harmful, draining your energy and blocking your ability to replenish. It is something you need to regulate because it is potentially harmful to your whole life being.

Grief affects the lungs and large intestine. The expression of grief is healthy and normal—it acknowledges what's going on inside you and within your life. By expressing grief, we are able to share with those around us the essential information regarding our mind-set, performance, and needs. Having our needs addressed helps us cope and rebalance faster and more smoothly. Uncontrolled grief, however, can sweep you downward into a gloom-filled worldview and out-of-control unhappiness. You know you have reached greater imbalance when sadness turns to listlessness and overall joyless living. Grief can lead to difficulties in breathing and a general heaviness throughout your body, especially in the area of your chest. You may also feel muscle aches and rigidity. Mind-body medicine maintains these imbalances, which can affect the large intestine with problems such as constipation or diarrhea. If you feel these symptoms, you will need to make it a priority to rebalance your energy.

Fear affects your kidneys and bladder, but fear is a necessity. Sometimes it is good to be afraid of that dark alley. Other times, our fear can serve as a prime motivator in getting ourselves the help we need to stay healthy or improve our performance. Yet at some point, you have to deal with your fear and let go. Fear arises spontaneously within the body and affects your well-being at all levels of body-mind-spirit. In its extreme, fear can weaken kidney functions, causing your energy to flow downward rather than upward. As a result, you may develop issues with frequent or involuntary urination. You may feel listless, sore, rigid, and antisocial. Panic (fast, sudden fright) generates violent palpitations and confusion. And fear, as discussed previously, blocks your higher quality energy, wreaking havoc on your focus and attention, and causing a wide range of other harmful energy effects on your body-mind-spirit.

Anger can have adverse affects on the liver and gallbladder, causing gas, indigestion, queasiness, and vomiting, as well as disrupting energy circulation throughout your body. Anger also brings about body aches and pains, a bad taste in the mouth, dizziness, and migraines. Yet anger is, as are your other emotions, a natural human feeling. Likewise, aggression (and feeling aggressive) is normal and healthy. It is, in fact, the driving force behind much goodness, creativity, and success. Anger, when mixed with positive aggression, can be the fire that lights your first steps (or if you are lucky, your whole path) toward eliminating a serious or potential obstacle in your life by aiming you in a more positive direction. The tricky part in dealing with aggression is that it is an energy that needs to be channeled positively or it can quickly flare up and get out of control.

The world of athletics is chock full of great examples of athletes who have used their anger and positive aggression to succeed. We have all seen the Olympic skier whipping down a white mountainside beautifully focused, making split-second adjustments, trying to outdo a previously disappointing performance. Or the tennis pro who, after missing more than one shot, comes back with what look like superhuman plays. By responding to anger in a balanced way, this emotional energy can be channeled into higher, smoother awareness, focus, and performance.

In contrast, we have all witnessed the opposite. The infamous story of Mike Tyson's ear-bite on Evander Holyfield in the WBA Boxing Championship provides a good example of aggression gone amuck.

Your job is to feel your emotions; you shouldn't ignore them. You don't necessarily have to put words to them, but you can simply try to feel them, experiencing their various energies and studying these energies—what they do for you and what messages they convey; how these energies translate into your thoughts and actions. By making yourself aware, you learn how to use the raw power of emotions to flow you toward specific areas of good and how to avoid various pitfalls.

The Informed Power of Emotional Memory

Most people say they can remember emotional events with sharp detail. This is because emotional events have a profound effect on your memory bank. Such memories also have an ongoing effect on the energetic quality and operations of your body, mind, and spirit, just as real-time emotions do.

In his 1951 book, *Organization and Pathology of Thought*, psychologist David Rapaport relates a compelling experiment originally written about in 1911 by French physician Édouard Claparède in his report titled "Recognition of Me-ness."[8]

As the story goes, Claparède had a patient—a forty-seven-year-old woman—who, similar to the character in the classic movie *Memento*, had apparently lost her ability to make new memories. One day, before his meeting with his patient, he carried out what he called a "curious experiment" to see if she could remember something that was purely emotional. He put a pin between his fingers and then, when they shook hands, he pushed the pin into her hand. She quickly pulled away, and in a few minutes, forgot that it happened. On the next occasion that he extended his hand for a shake, however, she swiftly withdrew hers and refused.

Claparède had witnessed and then written about two different types of memory: one type that stores events and experiences for conscious recollection at a later time, and another type of memory that can control your behavior without any learning—and without any awareness. Most important, this second memory storage can trigger powerful feelings, thoughts, and actions from under your radar.

The first memory bank is called *declarative memory*, which requires your conscious, intentional recall. As such, this kind of information involves conscious awareness and learning. If you touch a hot stove, you get burned; you "learn" not to touch it again, and you store that information in your memory to use for later. Declarative memory helps you see objects of your attention in full bloom; you see a wasp (like the one that stung you once before) as a wasp, not as a moth or housefly.

The second type of memory is *implicit memory*, which is virtually unconscious—you are not intentionally trying to recall the memory—and it is emotionally based, as evidenced when Claparède's patient refused to take his hand. This is the opposite of declarative memory and is sometimes called *procedural* (or *nondeclarative*) *memory*. Implicit memories, carrying procedural information and force, kick in automatically, like riding a bike or using a fork. Procedures that carry a great deal of emotional energy (such as giving someone the finger) fire so rapidly that they are completely unconscious, evident only in your actions or your reflections. In such cases, your brain doesn't just memorize a "task" and launch you into it; it combines with your instinctive fight-or-flight responses and makes a procedural value judgment at lightning speed—and then swiftly executes it, without ever consulting you. This is similar to what occurs with fear-based memory, which, as we discussed earlier, is fuzzy and inaccurate most of the time.

Implicit memory can be dangerous when combined with a negative mood and rapid changes in your blood chemistry. Under these circumstances, your judgment is impaired and strategic planning goes out the window, as they are replaced by reactivity. This not only messes up imminent (sometimes long-range) goals and causes energy drains at the physical level, but also shuts off the energy pipeline to your higher and spiritual mind. Such an imbalance can then launch you into a tail-spin of further trouble and create a negative loop of fear running under your awareness. When this happens, your mind associates new data with the original negative experience and adds that to your memory of it—all unconsciously.

For instance, the tone of your physician's voice when she is telling you that the results of your yearly blood testing look very good may trigger a fear response relating back to a time in your past—a time when someone using the same tone told you that things were all right when, in fact, they turned out catastrophically. You might even be thinking that your physician missed something or that the test was inaccurate. Such emotional prompts can be very hard to catch. If a companion were to ask later that day, "Why are you stressing over the results of your blood tests when they all came back normal?" you really may not know the answer. Nonetheless, this particular memory's energy consumption and influence on your thinking and behavior will continue until you identify it and learn to short-circuit it.

Of all harmful circuits, this is one of the worst because it stealthily invades positive moments of your life and accrues more negativity to reinforce itself, turning good times into bad and potential into liabilities. I recommend stepping back when you feel yourself becoming "hot" over relatively "cool" (innocuous) information before it is fully dispersed, or when you feel yourself becoming "hot" over information that should elicit a more pleasant response. This momentary pause gives you an opportunity to trace what's prompting you. By identifying the memory to which you have attached a current positive experience and that is negatively influencing your feelings about it, you can use your sense of reasoning to eliminate its stress. The more often you reverse this memory's influence when it bubbles up, the less future influence it will have on you. Eventually, you will be able to eliminate its influence altogether.

Another type of memory storage linked to emotional experiences is *flashbulb memory*. This kind of memory is associated with highly emotional, traumatic experiences. It is clear, crisp memory that includes not only major detail but secondary (or stray) detail as well. For example, if you were involved in a car accident, you may recall sideline details, such as how bright the sky was or certain scents and sounds—all with high resolution, photographic quality. This is why the scent of a certain cologne, a certain song on the radio, or the way autumn sunlight pours through a window in your house can reel your mind into the heart of an experience that occurred many years ago.

But flashbulb memory, as with other emotional memories, can fool you despite its sharpness of detail. This is because, many times, we add a narrative to the experience after the event—in part, depending on the point we want to make (e.g., in telling of a car accident, you may be trying to make the point that things happened very quickly but you were alert all the way; or that the road conditions were terrible; or if it weren't for your own expert driving, other cars may have been involved). So the details and memory evolve as a result of retelling them.

On a personal note, for me (as for most Americans), the story of the September 11, 2001, terrorist attack is powerful. I remember seeing images of the attack on television and then running to tell my wife. When I did, my memory was fairly accurate. But as I try to recall the original television footage now, I am no longer sure it is accurate. This is because, in the time since I saw the original images, I have seen a plethora of other images of the incident from many other angles and from many other reporting sources. I have discussed the incident with many different people and for many different reasons, using different details to make a variety of points. In short, I am no longer sure of the details I originally saw that morning on television. In situations like this, one's current memory draws more on a composite image of all the detail you have accrued since the original experience. Nonetheless, it is easy to think, *Yes, this is exactly the way I saw it*, when really, it probably isn't.

The importance of emotional memories doesn't center on accuracy; your brain's wiring doesn't seem to care much if your emotional memories are inaccurate 99 percent of the time. The one time they are right may, in fact, generate the life-saving reaction you need. It's no surprise that such emotional experiences continue to groove themselves deeper into your brain every time you remember them—orchestrating a cascade of chemicals that match the cascade they delivered the first time you lived through them.

In doing this, emotional memories energetically pull you into a negative energy feedback loop. Once you get sucked in, you are compromised at all energy levels of your body-mind-spirit. Your job is to practice identifying these memories, and limit or disengage the energetic effect(s) they may have on you and your life.

TRY THIS!

Next time you experience a spiraling mood, gently hold your hand over your heart and take a few deep and slow breaths. Then consider what you are about to do. Visualize the target of your activity: a person, place, or task (e.g., *I am in the middle of typing a report for work*). Think about how you are feeling. Don't put a name to it; feel into the emotion. Consider what "cool" (innocuous) information your mind and body are receiving. Take inventory. Is there a disjunction between anything you are feeling and your targeted activity? Visualize a former situation: identify how the disjunction between what you were feeling then and the goal of the situation might have impeded your performance. Ask yourself: *Are there things I do better when I feel this emotional energy? If so, what? What are my best options under this current of energy influence?*

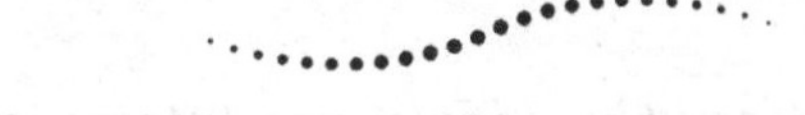

Mindfulness Is Your Emotional Key

In order to energetically change negative emotional patterns, you have to first be aware of them. However, awareness alone won't help much unless you also change your responses and behaviors. Nevertheless, the first step is awareness, and mindfulness is the way to become aware.

Tom, an engineer in his early forties, recently experienced an incident in which mindfulness could have saved him from experiencing a lot of negative emotions. He and his family were on vacation, and on his way out of their cabin after dinner, Tom picked up a book his wife had left on the picnic table and put it on her chair inside the veranda. Tom had enjoyed some wine with dinner, so his wife drove the family on a short coastal sightseeing tour as they looked for a place to get ice cream. The boys engaged in some humorous conversation in the back seat, and Tom's wife put on a CD of their favorite music. Detached and absorbed in his own mental space, Tom's mood turned sour. He could feel it rising like a fever in his body. His thoughts turned negative, and all he could think about were the family's finances—which he had gone over with his wife before they left for vacation so they could budget appropriately. Suddenly, words were pouring out of his mouth, and he was complaining about the family savings. This resulted in an argument between Tom and his wife, and left their sons concerned. Rather than relaxing and re-energizing the family, their after-dinner drive had turned into an energy drain and negative memory due to Tom's emotional reaction.

In the story above, Tom began to experience self-doubt, aggressive feelings of loathing, and other strong negative emotions that guided his actions. But you can train yourself to react differently through reflection. Applying this technique to Tom's situation, he would need to step back and ask:

- *What was happening just before my moment of emotional spiral?*
- *What was happening physically in my body?*
- *Can I identify the emotions I was experiencing?*
- *What thoughts came up for me and in what order?*
- *How did I react?*
- *What effect did my behavior have on others?*

By exploring these questions, Tom has the opportunity to examine the triggers for his negative and dysfunctional feelings and his flying off the handle. When he does, he will witness how his mood first started to shift from a holiday mood to a sour one when he noticed the book. Reflecting on the course of events, he can also witness that he immediately assumed his wife had just purchased the book, which wasn't part of their plan to stay on budget. When he calms and centers himself, he will feel in his gut that his reaction was over the top. But why?

As Tom looks more introspectively, he feels the aggressive energy starting in his body upon seeing the book, then thoughts of spending overbudget, then thoughts of a time years back when he and his wife had spent dangerously overbudget and it took months to recoup. But in going over the math in his head, he sees that this is not the case now. Why didn't he go over the math in his head earlier? Later on, he discovers that the book, the trigger for his emotional response, was something his wife had purchased a few years back.

In reflection, he witnesses the effect his behavior had on the rest of his family and wishes he could take it back. In the slower time of reflection, the unreasonableness of his behavior is clear to him. And in reflecting on what was happening just before the emotional spiral, he sees one other thing: the alcohol—though not excessive—was enough to impair his emotional reaction to the fear he has of overspending again. With further reflection in the days to come, he sees that his use of alcohol is part of his pattern of runaway emotions.

Mindfulness, at this phase, is observing and noting negative experiences sparked by shifts in mood and then describing or putting labels on the details that generated them. In order to do this, you need to learn to slow down your mind and step back from doing anything other than paying attention.

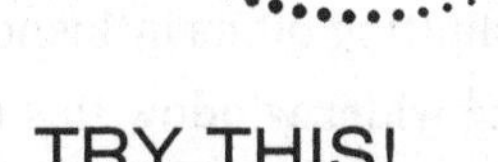

TRY THIS!

Set aside ten to fifteen minutes a day to practice mindfulness. Training for mindfulness is like any other life practice: most of your training is when you are not in the heat of the moment or the heat of actual battle, so that you are ready when you need it. When you were young, you practiced riding a bike in a parking lot so that by the time you rode your bike on the street, you were ready. Mindfulness works similarly—practice when you don't need it so that when you need it, it is there!

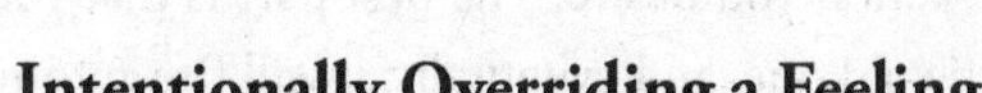

Intentionally Overriding a Feeling

As you become aware of the energy of dysfunctional feelings you experience in specific circumstances, you can begin to intentionally override them and the negative effect they have on your thoughts, actions, and feelings in that situation. Again, mindfulness is the key.

You can begin to regulate these feelings by making yourself mindful of natural pauses within important moments of action in which strategic considerations are made. Give yourself a heads up before these situations so you can be sensitive to when strategic moments appear. Our aim is to practice slowing down, blocking the influence of negative emotions, increasing your awareness of the situation, feeling into your choices, and considering your best response.

As you learn to block the influence of certain emotions that get in the way, the next time you are in that given situation, that particular emotion (its informed power) will have less influence on you. This gives you a bigger window with which to consciously choose differently. With each time you practice shutting off its influence, it will begin to have less and less effect. Using the wider window this regulation offers, your job is then to detach and give yourself a broad, more relaxed perspective. This offers you a chance to take inventory of your internal and external environments.

As you do this, try to understand and feel more into the energy of the situation, using it to consider and strategize your next move. You can even use your mind to charge yourself with the appropriate balancing energy before responding. For example, you can think of a song or visualize a photo you have been using to train your mind to calm. What's key is that you have already trained with these tools. Now trained, your mind will provide you good and fast help automatically. This will, in turn, enable you to create new circuits that operate in accordance with the energy and action you desire. The best part is that your new circuit will short out the old one, and eventually, it will fire automatically.

Use the Informed Power of Association

Once you know those situations that tend to energetically lead you to negative emotional reactions (as well as those that link to positive ones) and you have started to take advantage of the natural pauses within them, I encourage you to start using mindfulness not only to divert harmful feelings but to self-regulate and replace them with the appropriate ones.

You can, for example, use the energy of music or natural sound and the positive emotion(s) you associate with these to get ready for an important situation. (Or you can use guided imagery, or combinations of sound and imagery.) Use these to raise and balance your psychic and physical energy so your responses will be more optimized. As a result, you also use energy to train your mind to identify and attach more quickly to positive—rather than negative—details within a given situation the next time around, and all the times after.

Just imagine the difference it would make if you took one whole month to replace only one daily, dysfunctional emotional response. And what if you replaced another the next month and continued disarming the harmful energetic effects of negative emotions one month at a time? Imagine how much sharper your daily thoughts, actions, and spirit would be by the end of just six months. Imagine the amount of stress you could end within a year, and how much healthier and happier you could live! Let that be your incentive.

You can learn to identify your energetic triggers by paying attention to the natural cues and rewards within any given situation. Simply make yourself aware: *I did "such and such" and it served me well.* For instance, an orchestra musician may learn that if she replaces her need for peer approval with staying interested in the composition she is playing, she performs better; and that spreads to the whole orchestra. As was discussed earlier, the first step to accomplishing this is mindfulness. With this in mind, begin by paying attention to how specific people, places, and things affect you—even in the slightest ways. This will enable you to discover what sparks the emotions that guide you to positive outcomes.

The Energy of Conflicting Emotions

Sometimes we experience conflicting feelings within ourselves. Although these conflicts can and should be dealt with, being sensitive to them offers opportunities in terms of self-discovery, and can help you determine how to best use your energy in order to achieve those things that make you happiest and healthiest.

Consider an individual who, on the outside, seems to have everything in the world going for him; yet he complains that he feels incomplete or worse. Or he cannot feel satisfied with his accomplishments, so he keeps chasing more and more of them, never taking the time to enjoy what he has.

Or take another individual who has just accomplished something she has desired for quite some time. This can be anything from running a marathon to getting a promotion at work. But for some reason, her delight is short lasting. Why is it that satisfaction sometimes only lasts for a few hours and then begins to wane rapidly? Next thing you know, excitement drains and is replaced with lower energy.

This emotional pattern typically happens as a result of an attachment to energy that is not connected to the cultivation of one's higher Self. Many times, such attachments are more connected to outside influences than to the accomplishments that nourish the very core of who we are. Your mind feels the difference between the two; our bodies feel the difference. So feeling that conflict can be a wake-up call to get things on a better track.

When an accomplishment is connected to a core need (a necessity to evolve your highest mind to the next rung on the ladder) achieving it resonates throughout your whole being. In other words, you feel great physically, mentally, and spiritually. You maintain this energy, and it fuels you through the next step in the evolution of your full life being. Asian medical and philosophical traditions view this pattern as your primary life purpose. In fact, they maintain that attending to this pattern helps you move toward all other goals and happiness.

Sometimes negative and dysfunctional emotional energies get the better of us (particularly fears or the need to please). In these cases, we may switch paths from what we need to be doing and, instead, strive for something that isn't in line with our deeper Self—something that offers safety or addresses another immediate emotional need. As a result, we may experience conflicting feelings about what we are doing. Some people go to college, for instance, to earn a degree because it is the path that will yield the quickest employment, or because their chosen field is based on what someone else thinks they do best. Following college, this individual finds employment in the field he is trained for, perhaps in a location that he didn't have in mind, and his life begins to drift further and further from the needs of his deeper Self. This imbalance shuts off the essential higher-quality energy line, leaving him feeling drained and potentially dissatisfied. The disparity between his inner and outer worlds is the source of his mixed feelings. Outwardly, he may appear to have it all, but inwardly, he feels like something is missing. Something is.

Imagine if you could see movies of the decisive personal moments in your life that have contributed to the places you have been and where you are now. What would you see? A person I know recently did this. He found himself lamenting that, in hindsight, he could see just how easily he could have accomplished his most important life goals—those most connected with his deeper Self and heartfelt dreams. Yet in the "real time" of his life, he now saw that he frequently took the more difficult path—the energy-consuming path.

Options often pop up more clearly in retrospect. This man is not alone in this experience—most of us have experienced such feelings. On the other hand, there is no time like the present to start experiencing life differently.

To this end, become objective in "real time" by looking at your life choices with a cooled down, *detached mind-set.* Through detachment, you become more objective, slowing down the urgency for reaction and simultaneously checking in with the needs of your inner Self; you scan for the smoothest, most satisfying course of action. When you see the connection between what you surround yourself with and what you do, and how that relates to deeper personal needs, you tend to feel more at peace and you experience more satisfaction. You also can navigate your life with more confidence and skill.

Today especially, too many individuals are aiming a lot of their attention toward a less functional (and lower quality energy) direction of the material world. You can certainly learn things about yourself by exploring the external world. It's fun to be on the run and experiencing new people, places, and things—no one is saying don't do that. But if you are looking for your Self (the headquarters of your consciousness) out there at the energy level of material accomplishment, you run a high risk of not finding what you are looking for.

Self does not energetically exist in this physical realm. So by chasing externally driven desires, you are, in essence, chasing someone else's dream (or worse, a media-driven dream that isn't even real) and losing touch with who you really are—your own unique life purpose and energy. This disconnection leaves you feeling drained and perhaps unhealthy—instead of energetic, healthy, and beautiful. You may feel your life needs deeper meaning or lacks meaning altogether. The good news is that you can feel the conflict, and by becoming aware, you can change course to reverse the negative moods that arise.

To avoid having an external, low-grade energy powering and informing your mind, you must prioritize spending time to explore your Self inwardly. Then you can train your mind to identify the external things that truly resonate with your entire life being. Subsequently, this energy (force and information) will begin to shape your reality *for* you.

To do anything else to "find your Self" is a diversion as well as an energy-consuming enterprise. It could be likened to spending your time and energy on finding land for a structure you want to build; hiring an architect to design the building; working to pay for it all; and then, after all is said and done, asking yourself what you think you might do with the building you have built. Most of us wouldn't do such a thing. But many people live that way and then wonder why life is, at times, difficult and not all that satisfying. When they look back, they have mixed feelings. But it doesn't have to be that way. Better to be aware of those mixed feelings in the present. The question is: Are you ready to do things differently when you feel them? It's never too late, and the energy you need is always available.

When Your Emotions Conflict with Other People's

When you feel emotionally conflicted with other people (or yourself), it can be very energy consuming, eating into other things you do. You can use reason to sort out the way you are feeling, but not right away; you need to acknowledge your feelings first.

Successful conflict resolution starts with rational data but doesn't ignore the world of feelings and emotions. However, feelings that are generated from powerful influences that can have their roots in your past can run under your radar, and may not always be manageable through rational thinking. So at first, you may need to let yourself feel into the emotions that arise from the situation. As we have said, you don't have to name them. But try to understand their characteristics by feeling their effects on your body, mind, and spirit.

Ask yourself: *What are the messages of my emotions and those of others—to me and to them?* Don't be afraid to confront these. Some people would rather avoid this confrontation, but that will only add more tension and cause you further problems down the line.

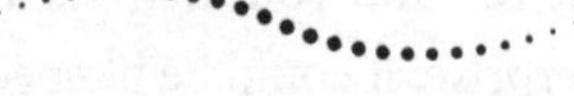

TRY THIS!

Next time you sense conflict between yourself and another individual, take a moment and make yourself aware. Feel the conflicting emotions emanating from both of you. Stay cool and try the following:

- Visualize yourself in the conflicting situation. Consider the other individual(s) involved. Visualize what happened (events, conversations) to set off these emotional responses.
- Put yourself in the other person's mind. Consider what assumptions that individual may be making about the situation.
- See the situation from the perspective of the peripheral people involved, and consider how they feel about the conflict and about each other. See how they may have tried to deal with it. If they have not, consider why. What assumptions might they be making?

A good look at what's going on can help you understand the irrational, emotional forces that are adding to tensions. Use your reasoning to feel into the energies of each of these perspectives before responding. If you rely on logic right off the bat, you might (and probably will) only fuel the fires.

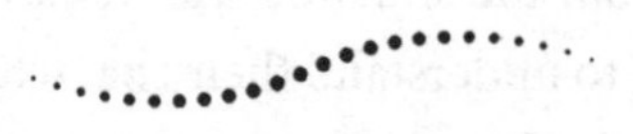

Healing a Broken Heart

You may be feeling or know someone who is feeling the emotional pain of a broken heart. One thing you don't want to do is trigger memories of times and places that remind you of the breakup. Instead, it works well to alter your mind-set with the energy of safe times, such as those you experienced in your childhood. To do this, you might listen to funny children's songs that you enjoyed when you were young. Or you might watch a film or read a story that amused you as a child. It may sound silly, but tapping into the energy of humor in any of these formats can really work.

You don't need to limit yourself to items from your childhood, however. As with any other type of informed power, it's about tapping into the type that is right for you in your particular situation.

One individual I know was feeling so lousy after a breakup that he took numerous, proactive steps to reverse his harmful moods. As a first step, he determined that one of his happiest times was when he used to hang out with his hockey buddies in college. On their way to games, they would blast "Eye of the Tiger" by Survivor to pump themselves up. He then painted his apartment new and brighter colors, and he put posters on the walls that reminded him of a place in New York's Adirondack Mountains where he and his parents used to camp when he was a child. He also put up pictures of the lake where he and his father used to fish.

This regimen worked wonders. In fact, it put him into the same kind of good mood he felt back when he was younger and actively doing these things. He discovered that every time he played "The Eye of the Tiger" now or spent time enjoying the pictures, his mind would stop obsessing on his relationship. He put the song on his iPod and started playing it several times a day as a soundtrack to a slide show he'd made from the pictures, especially when he could feel himself reminiscing about his partner. This gave him instant relief, and he started feeling better and better with each day. For the next month or so, whenever he felt his mind derailing and being pulled into the emotional quicksand of his breakup, he'd play his song. This helped get him back on track and soothed him through this delicate broken-heart phase. It also helped rebuild his energy to the point where he could add other energy elements to continue the healthy trajectory.

Self-Destructive Moods

If you are so sad or angry that you are in a self-destructive mood, you can use the energies of art and your natural environment to lift you up. Sometimes, when people are feeling the overwhelming pressures of work, a relationship, or a goal, they begin to panic. This state of mind can make a person feel like giving up, which can lead to harmful remedies and reckless behaviors. When individuals enter this panicky state, they intentionally (or unintentionally) subject themselves to energies (people, places, things, and activities) that amplify the fast frequencies of their panic. For example, this occurs when a frazzled person spends time around an angry friend or goes on a drinking binge. These tendencies make your energy more dysfunctional. The best solution is to step back and activate your brain's emotional systems. Decide what kind of emotional energy you need to rebalance in a particular situation. So if you are angry, you will need to send your mind slower, calming emotional frequencies to help you rebalance your feelings.

Dealing with Negative Emotions Whether You Are an Introvert or Extrovert

The trick, whether you see yourself as an introvert or an extrovert, is in keeping your emotions balanced with the energy you need at different points in your day.

To this end, a challenge for the introvert stems from your usual comfort zone, which is internal. When your head isn't clear and is, in fact, causing or adding to a negative mood, you need a break. This may mean getting out of your head for a while.

One way to do this is to find your way into the flow of an external activity. The good news: even though your activity is external you can still get into a flowing mind-set—in a comfy, more private zone. Creative and intellectual endeavors, such as playing an instrument or writing, work well to get and keep you flowing. Be sure to stay with your activity until you rebalance. As you do this, take care not to attach to any negative triggers that activate your negativity. Additionally, you want to avoid expecting the popularly established "external signs" that you are feeling better, such as being talkative and boisterous. For you, falling into those traps can drain energy and drive you into further negativity.

Getting into and sustaining your psychic flow, whether you are an introvert or an extrovert, will eliminate or bypass the information that has been pulling you into a negative mood and consuming your energy. As your good energy goes up, your negative mood goes away. This is the energy loop that you want to restore positivity and check negativity at the door.

The general challenge for extroverts is different, however. It may require you to stay aware of your attraction to outside distractors that won't resolve your negative mood—e.g., going on a road trip, vacation, or robust socializing. One extrovert I know told me that his way of curing his depressions is "party, party, party." Yet he admits that "as soon as the party is over, the next wave of depression hits." If you are an extrovert, be aware of this energy trap, as it can consume more energy than it will deliver.

Whether you are an introvert or an extrovert, the more you practice daily meditation, the easier it is for you to stay positive when confronted with negative triggers. One possible reason for this is that you have learned and practiced your ability to regularly activate that place in your mind that enables you to turn off certain mental tendencies and urgencies (frequencies and chemistries), and turn on others instead. This allows you to block dysfunctional energetic influences from your own emotional narratives and memories, or from outside influences and individuals. Again, if you have practiced meditation and mindfulness, you can better clear these influencers. So don't wait to get into a mood swing to begin practicing. Start today.

Predict Your Emotional Energy Needs

Certain pieces of art—music, painting, photography, film—that you have "a craving for" can help you forecast the type of energy you will need in the coming days. Yet just because you are inclined toward a certain piece art doesn't mean that its type of energy is going to be good for you. For example, you may be inclined to fuel yourself with edgy music and angry lyrics. If you are on your way to participate in an athletic event, that formula may deliver just the energy you need. However, if you are listening to the same piece while on your way to a meeting with your boss over next year's contract—and you already feel irritated about the details—this energy may launch inappropriate feelings and behaviors.

Art can help you become more self-aware. Use a current attraction to a certain type of art to learn more about your mind-set as well as predict where you are going emotionally and behaviorally. Use the art to tell you what energy you need to stay in balance. Remember our discussion of yin-yang: you will find your balance by complementing with the opposite energy. If you are angry and attracted to aggressive art, step back and consider what tasks you have imminently coming up. If this energy is appropriate, when you feel you have maximized its benefits, look toward more calming energies before your aggression goes overboard and becomes damaging. If you are sad and attracted to melancholy tunes, again, step back and assess. If this energy is not a match with upcoming tasks, look toward something uplifting.

When you find yourself attracted to a certain piece of art, ask yourself about the piece and the message it is conveying. Consider whether the message pertains to you or to future endeavors, and think about whether you need more or less of the energy the art is giving to you. If you cannot use the feelings it provokes to your advantage, consider what energy *can* give you an advantage.

Use the strong, informed power of the art to guide you to where you are headed, and use visualization to see yourself already in your best energetic state, acting confidently, in control, and flowing. The more brain areas you use, the more amplified the energetic effect.

Once you have considered your best state, think about how a change in your mood can help you achieve it. Psychologically, whatever mood you generate will call forth other thoughts and memories to increase it. Choose the best mood, and it will shower you with the best match with what you want to happen next.

This kind of pre-emptive thinking will take you off a potentially harmful track toward your goals and put you on a more energetically constructive one.

Improving a Mood Together

Just as a negative mood can spiral into more negativity, good feelings can attract more good feelings. This is why you can use the energy of mutually positive emotional memories to improve a negative mood both you and your partner may be going through. All you have to do is take any positive experience the two of you have shared—the more exciting the better—and make some energy medicine of it.

For example, if you have video footage of a vacation you took together back when you first met, you can use it to create a montage. Try adding some of your mutually enjoyed music as a soundtrack—perhaps a song from your wedding or from when you first started dating—and make a short video using some of the vacation footage. The combined energies of visuals and sound will not only spike the positive influencing power of each, but will also unite you into the positive frequencies and chemistries from earlier in your relationship.

One husband used film from an ocean sunrise he and his wife watched on holiday when they spontaneously got engaged. His soundtrack was "These Are the Days" by 10,000 Maniacs, a band his wife loves, and whose music he learned about and loves through her. Their music—and this song in particular—went everywhere with them in their early days. He used his creation to relieve a negative mood that had invaded their relationship. When his wife experienced the film and her husband's brightened spirits, her own irritations began to fade. The experience put smiles on both of their faces, and their hearts warmed together.

Make Virtuous Memory

I recently met a colleague on a walk. It was a lovely spring day, and we were both relaxing outside the research center where we work. We walked a bit and talked about how the high energy of spring was especially welcome this year, after the harsh, cold, and snowy winter we had experienced in the Northeast. We spoke about our respective research. He asked me how I was doing, and I said that I was enjoying immersing myself in research because so much of it deals with just feeling and living nicer.

"Honestly," I said, "looking back over my career so far—and not to sound platitudinous—the parts I remember most are the days when I was able to put a piece of information out there, and it helped somebody feel better or healthier or more spirited . . . the days when I really connected with someone."

"There is nothing platitudinous about it," he replied. "That's the way it is for me too."

As we have discussed, honesty, compassion, acceptance, peace, and unconditional love are the Virtues (characteristics) of the Universe. Their energies are the energy characteristics of our own original being.

By making new memories of behaviors in which you are acting in Virtue, you create a storage tank of emotional energy to fuel you whenever you need to shift into greater positivity.

Exercises and Practices

1. Decide what type of energy you need to balance at the moment. Put on a piece of music or use a piece of visual art that can deliver that frequency and message. Place yourself into a meditative mind-set, and make yourself mindful within all three levels of consciousness: lower mind, higher mind, and spiritual mind. Be there for a while. Then place your awareness into your highest mind (spiritual); and meditate on the virtues of honesty, compassion, acceptance, peace, and unconditional love. Use your emotional memory to see yourself in experiences that present each of these Virtues. If you wish, you can also (or instead) create new scenarios in which you see yourself employing these Virtues in encounters with people you know. Breathe in slowly and deeply. Feel into each scenario as though you are looking through a gold-colored lens so that everything has a bright golden sheen. Now inhale the whole image, slowly and deeply. Take a few more in-breaths. Luxuriate in the energy.

2. The next time you are feeling bored and burnt out, instead of lying back, push the pedal to the metal. Switch tasks to something more deeply rewarding. Feel yourself flow again.

3. Spend a day trying to see the positive side of everything.

7

USING ENERGY TO REVERSE CONFLICT

Every time you don't follow your inner guidance,
you feel a loss of energy, loss of power,
a sense of spiritual deadness.

—Shakti Gawain

The ability to feel conflict is essential. This capacity is wired into all of us so that we know when something isn't quite right—when we are in a state of imbalance. We rely on this sensation (energy) to stay healthy in body, mind, and spirit, so conflict is, in this way, unavoidable. And not all conflict should be seen as harmful. Much of its effect depends on your perceptive lens and in how you respond to it. As with negative emotions, it is your response to conflict that determines how it will affect you.

Conflict, at best, gives you the opportunity to develop new perspectives, insights, and techniques for making corrections and rebalancing. In many ways, it is as the philosopher Nietzsche said: "Whatever doesn't destroy you will make you stronger." From vaccines to strength training to unraveling the mysteries of science, conflict can lead to tremendous new growth and success. It can take you places you never imagined. But for this to happen, you almost always need to make yourself receptive to the possibility for positive change.

The silver lining to the challenges of conflict is self-evolution and the cultivation of higher energy at all levels of body, mind, and spirit.

Your Response Is Your Choice

You have the freedom to treat conflict in a positive way—you have choice. When you feel conflict coming on, you can train yourself to step back, take a good look at what's happening externally and within, and make the necessary corrections to bring yourself back to a point of balance. You can walk away from your conflicts stronger and healthier. As a result, you can also know more about yourself, others, and the world around you.

On the other hand, the energy of conflict can guide you to extreme dysfunction—an individual, interpersonal, and goal-oriented level—if you let it. Unattended, the energy of unmanaged conflict will generate harmful consequences, including distraction, confusion, and depression, and can lead to all kinds of physical and mental health problems. It can create gridlock in your life and steer you into inappropriate life choices. Consequently, everyone needs to manage their conflicts in order to stay on track with life goals.

I knew a young man who, straight out of college, began a teaching career in a junior high school. He was bright, well educated, and quite social. He also possessed a lot of motivation and was willing to "walk the extra mile."

Nonetheless, every day on the job was riddled with conflict for him. It would start with conflict with students, which led to conflict with parent; other teachers; and finally, his administrators. In the end, he was let go from his teaching position. He took another teaching job, but it soon followed the same path. The conflicts he felt worsened. He reported waking up mornings and not wanting to even get out of bed, much less go to work. There were times almost every day when his conflicts with students were so bad he would close his eyes mid-discussion, and see himself walking out the door and never coming back. During these times, he frequently became ill with colds and had trouble with fatigue, insomnia, and digestive issues.

To soothe himself, he began having a few beers with dinner—then more. This grew into other problems, including unwanted weight gain, fuzzy thinking on the days after drinking, and even lower energy in the evenings, which meant he was unable think about what he needed to do to resolve his conflicts. He went from fulltime teacher to substitute in order to keep bread on the table. He experienced similar problems with this part-time employment. Nonetheless, he continued it for over a year before realizing that his conflicts weren't going away—he was, in fact, bringing them along with him. And now they'd expanded to include a rocky relationship in which he later felt trapped—a relationship that consumed his energy to the point that he felt mentally paralyzed and physically ill most of the time.

Up until then, his primary drives had been competition and outcome. He measured himself against what others had achieved externally, and was not satisfied until he had the perception that he had either matched or surpassed them. His self-esteem depended on how he measured into this comparison. All this affected the quality of his energy, as well as his physical and mental and spiritual health.

Not until he started making choices that began to nurture the cultivation of his innermost Self did his conflicts start to retract. These decisions began with taking more time to introspect and understand his true nature, and whether his desire to teach was rooted in who he really is or if it was coming from somewhere else—somewhere dysfunctional. Putting your focus on Self is at the core of resolving dysfunctional conflict and rebalancing into a better place.

To manage conflict successfully, it is first essential to understand what is really going on—to you, around you, and within you. There isn't a one-size-fits-all formula to resolution; each conflict has contributing factors. You must appreciate each conflict's specific roots—externally and internally—and see how these factors apply to you. Somewhere in the mix is your unique and full life being, and that must come into account. If you deny this introspection, your conflict will return until you do look at the whole picture or you damage your attentional network's capability to do so—which will lead to more serious problems.

What's Driving You?

People are driven by reason and by emotions that can be irrational.

For example, a person may come off as having a my-way-or-the-highway attitude, acting as if no one should do anything that differs from his way. His behavior may seem egotistical to certain individuals around him, and they may respond to him as though their conclusion that he is ego driven is accurate—yet it may not be so at all. In fact, it could be just the opposite. He may be driven by a torrent of emotions rooted in his own unconscious insecurity, which could, in turn, be rooted in a myriad of circumstances. Perhaps he was raised by a prejudicial, domineering father who regularly withheld love, compliments, and acknowledgment. Now this individual's hurt feelings about being unrecognized by his father are unconsciously encouraging him to strategize ways to micro-control people and situations in his life. For him, his drive toward such behavior has become procedural (automatic) and happens under his radar, in a virtual instant. Energetically, this habit to microcontrol kicks in at work, when he's out with friends or family—everywhere. It is at the root of many of his conflicts and stress; it consumes large amounts of his daily energy as he reasons out ways to exert control on his surroundings. This need is what guides his tendency to overwork in most settings, especially—and ironically—where his efforts are least appreciated. This procedural pattern is what prevents him from sufficiently re-energizing by tapping into higher quality energy. And his attachment to this pattern sustains the feeling of conflict in his life, interfering with his health and happiness.

Feelings, which are playing under your radar like this and are deeply grooved into your emotional memory, can be very powerful and difficult to manage—especially when they are rooted in past experience. With some assistance, however, and greater self-awareness, we may be able to better understand how they work. The hope is that such awareness and understanding will lead to better regulation, less stress, and smoother rebalancing.

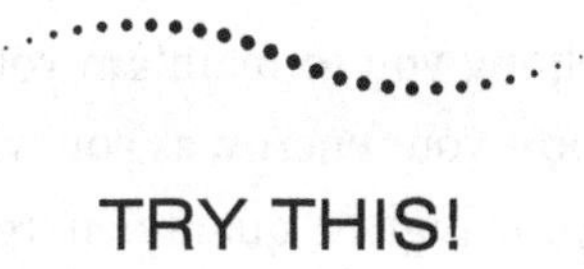

TRY THIS!

Think back to a conflict. Step back, keeping your mind and heart open. Mindfully look into the situation. Consider what was at stake for you and for others. Visualize what changes occurred in the scenario as it was unraveling that launched the conflict in the first place. Visualize what actions you attempted to take to deal with the conflict. Consider how others felt about the conflict. Consider any actions you might have taken that may have led to a better resolution.

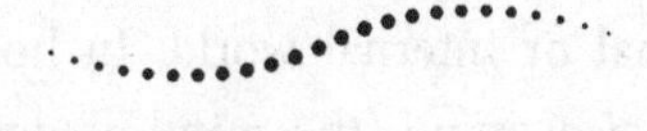

Compassionate Listening

Compassionate listening involves paying attention to all points of view without judgment. This is difficult most of the time because we are often thinking of what we are going to say next (especially in rebuttal) to someone before they have even finished speaking. Sometimes our response is to a point they are not even going to make. We usually don't know when we have done this because we are not listening; this behavioral habit closes us off to important information we need to accurately access what is being communicated to us.

So your first step toward more compassionate listening is to appreciate and practice listening more fully—with an open mind and heart. The next step is to make yourself aware of any irrational thoughts and feelings that may be bubbling up inside you and keeping you in conflict. Say no to these. Turn them off like a switch. As you listen, you can more easily identify your best and most advantageous response for all. Through compassionate and honest listening, this will become abundantly clear to you, helping you to maintain your good energy instead of draining it. It will boost your energy, as you will flow in sync with the Universal Virtue and your highest quality energy. Like magic, you will see how much more positive you and those around you feel. This helps formulate smooth and functional conflict resolution, inwardly and externally, and creates new positive energy feedback loops as rewards toward future application.

Learn to Identify the Informed Power of an Attached Mind

As we have discussed, you feel conflict as you begin to resist various things in your external or internal world. In holistic psychology, we believe that the *biological mind* (the mind associated with the body) electrochemically attaches to what we like and resists those things we don't like. We further believe that the *untrained mind*—a mind that is constantly allowed to attach this way—is the root of conflict and much energy drain. The remedy is self-regulation.

Self-regulation begins with truthfully seeing who you are. The way to do this is to connect with your original nature (highest mind). This nature is characterized by the original energy nature of the Universe, and the way to connect with it is to cultivate the energy of Virtue and live in accordance to the principle of yin-yang. For instance, as you expend energy with reason or analysis, you can provide balance by periodically shifting your attention to creative and spiritual thoughts (such as compassion, acceptance, honesty), and to activities that replenish you and keep you flowing. The most powerful tools we presently have to help with balance are meditation, visualization, reflection, and the sensory activities with which we can augment these.

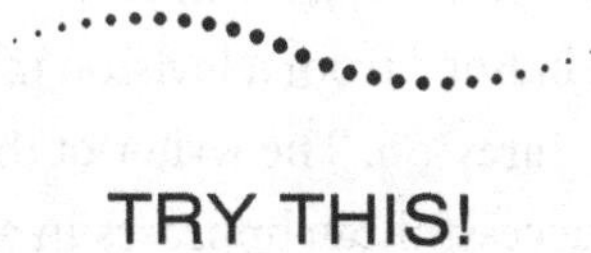

TRY THIS!

Next time you are in conflict with someone, as soon as you feel the first signs of conflict, tell yourself that your mind has attached to something and is out of flow. Making sure your mind is not attached is important to unblocking your energies and targeting your focus toward resolving conflict. Repeating this step every time you feel the very first buzz of conflict helps you start identifying your pattern of attachment and conflict earlier and faster.

After you've recognized the conflict, step back and take a breath. Use reflection, center yourself, and feel into your highest mind. Then ask yourself: *Is this the way of my highest Self? Is my highest Self guiding me or is something else guiding me? Am I feeling, thinking, and acting in accordance with Virtue? Am I acting in balance and harmony?* If not, tell yourself it is the energy of whatever your mind is attaching to that is guiding you. See if you can identify what it is. Let the feeling of conflict pass through you, and let go of it. Then use a technique, such as visualization, to reboot—because you are in an energy-draining and blocking mode.

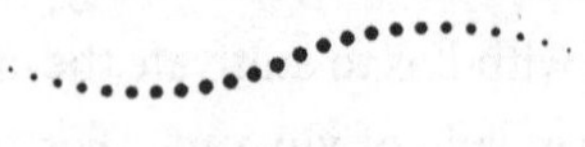

Wired to Resist

No doubt, you have noticed that it is easy to resist something or someone that goes against your beliefs or pre-existing loyalties. But why is it so easy to resist something or someone? And why can we get pretty aggressive about it—and fast?

There was an iconic television commercial that aired before cigarette commercials were banned from television in 1971. This ad was for a brand of smokes called Tareyton. The writer of the commercial came up with one of the most successful catchphrases in advertising history: "Us Tareyton smokers would rather fight than switch."[1] In the commercial, the anthem humorously communicated that the smoker, who revealed a black eye, would not be switching his brand of cigarette—at least not without a fight.

The slogan itself, however, may have nailed the workings of the human mind more accurately than the writers could have known at the time. With the benefits of today's powerful imaging instruments, we are able to see that humans are literally wired to resist and even attack anything with which we disagree—whether that "thing" is a tiger in the bushes or a concept. And we usually disagree with anything that is not our own brand—our own way of doing things. This is why, when we are in conflict with people, we think that we are (of course) in the right and the other person is (of course) in the wrong. We all do this. On a personal note, after spending thirty-five years in higher education, I have never met a student who was in conflict with one of his professors (or a colleague with another colleague) who thought that the other person was the one who was right. Sometimes we get pretty aggressive about maintaining our stand. Just consider the world of politics and political issues.

Early Energy Signs of Conflict

As we hear others speak, our minds open to incoming information. Then our minds narrow, as we hear and attach onto the things we want to hear and fight against the things we don't want to hear.

We may sometimes react with anger as well—in proportion to how much we oppose what we are hearing. This reaction can easily spiral into more negativity, some of it being guided by unconscious attachments and procedures from our present or past. When this happens, a conflict can turn to wildfire—very quickly.

Stopping this wildfire begins with recognition and being mindful. However, our tendency to attach to particular people and ideas is not the only early energy sign of conflict we need to be aware of. From the perspective of holistic medicine, we believe there are several sources of conflict that can derail us from a flow state and initiate anxiety and struggle. However, these distractions, irrational thoughts, and destructive behaviors also provide early cues to help in self-regulation. So your continued practice of mindfulness will be key in identifying and managing these cues.

Although these sources come in many forms, a few are frequently involved in causing conflict. For example, you might attach to a feeling that you deserve acknowledgment, reward, or certain action from someone, or some organization or institution. When you do not get the response your mind wants, this creates conflict.

Conflict is also created when you attach to the view that another person, an organization, or an institution is being inflexible, disrespectful, self-righteous, questionable, dishonest, or egotistical. Conflict may also stem from attaching to a negative emotion such as anger toward someone, an organization, or an institution. This negative emotion may even evolve into an attachment to the desire for difficulty, loss, or harm to befall someone. Furthermore, conflicts often result from attaching to certain misunderstandings, particularly when you allow your mistaken beliefs to guide you.

Each of these conditions can cause or further conflict as well as consume your energy; and at the same time, block higher energy resources, and your ability to stop your energy drain and replenish.

Harmful Passivity

Some people become energetically passive when in conflict—an approach that may cover up an intentional personal preference for fighting. Or it may be rooted in passivity from the individual's confusion over just what to do in a tense situation and in their inability to regulate a conflict to a better result.

Either way, dealing with conflict passively leads to more and bigger problems personally and interpersonally. And the result is further irritation, anxiety, and at times, loss of the healthy self-esteem you need to get things done and feel good about yourself.

Passivity can also result in a misunderstanding or a lack of good information. People in such circumstances tend to feel anxious and can consequently channel energy into further conflict, competition, or fighting.

Overcompensating to avoid confrontation in the name of compassion and understanding can also further conflict rather than dissolve it. Truth, honesty, and positive aggression (compassionate firmness) are often needed to get all the important information on the table; flexibility can, all along the way, be more soothing, leading to greater self- and interpersonal discovery, as well as peaceful and harmonious resolution.

Stopping Conflict

As I've been saying, when you find yourself in conflict, before you do another thing, step back and tell yourself firmly: *This is my mind attaching.*

Be aware that you may, in fact, like what you are thinking, saying, or doing. After all, it provides you with a vent, and that can formulate its own reward loop. But that doesn't mean you should allow it to continue. In the end, you may be rewarding yourself for sustaining and even heightening the conflict.

You also need to be aware that the more you attach to negative prompts, the more they will ingrain, the faster they will trigger each subsequent time, and the faster you will lose and block your life's essential energies. It is thus important to recognize right away that your mind is stuck in a *conditioned response.* This is electrochemical turbulence, and it is not your true Self.

Once you have recognized this, take a step back and let go of your conditioned response. This is your opportunity to put the best "you" forward—the "you" that you consciously approve of, and that is evolving in accordance with your full living being and your life purpose. In addition, it is your opportunity to harmonize with others. You know the feeling of flow—when you are completely absorbed, interested, focused, and happy. And you know the feeling of turning off a particular energy. Switch off the negative energy, and use your subtle energy tools of reflection or visualization to ease you into a flowing mind again.

Of course, the more energy tools you have prepared and practiced in advance, the more effective they will be for you now. Similarly, you must train yourself to start identifying every time you are feeling this way. Make yourself mindful that you have attached to one of these areas of conflict, and that this is energetically guiding and sustaining your struggle.

Remember one of the key themes of body intelligence: the core of self-regulation is Self and self-awareness. This is the vantage point from which you can identify your full life being's genuine needs and its power. As such, you need to periodically ask yourself what you need from any situation—and in this case, those in which you feel conflicted.

As you check in with yourself, you can separate needs from the wants or desires your mind is attaching to. Avoid irrational thinking. Most important, keep your mind open, stay in flow, and regulate your actions within your best interests.

Once you are back in a flowing mind-set, it is also important to listen to what the other individual is saying. Use reason to help you understand them. As you do, sync your body and mind with your true Self, Virtue, and the principle of yin-yang. Finally, respond with honesty, compassion, acceptance, peace, and unconditional love. (I'll repeat these lines again in the coming pages. I hope they become a mantra for you.)

One interesting thing I love about the way the mind works is that all of these behaviors are energetically catching to others. This means that those you are in conflict with can literally catch some of your positivity.

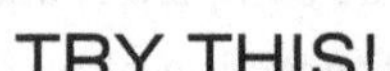

TRY THIS!

The next time you feel that you are about to enter a conflict, follow the instructions to halt it in its tracks. It is important to catch a potential conflict before it starts so that you can avert it. As we have said, being mindful of the early signs of conflict will help you do this. Consider whether you are attaching to something that is preventing you from finding peaceful solutions. Once you have identified your conflict, let go of these attachments and go back to your flowing mind. Then listen to the other individual, and use reason to help you understand them. Respond with authenticity, peace, and compassion.

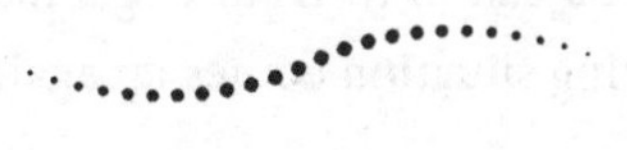

Moving Past Conflict

Sometimes, the conflict cannot be resolved, in which case the lesson is to accept that fact and move on. This is often difficult—we get caught up in proving that we are right at any cost—but if you are checking in with your Self and simultaneously looking outwardly, you can more reasonably move forward. Similarly, in the dojo, the mindful martial artist learns that after all is said and done, her sparring opponents are really her partners.

Just as sparring opponents help train each other to higher skill, greater happiness, and higher consciousness, you also have the opportunity to cultivate your full life being to a higher-quality energy state every time you experience and deal with conflict. This is conflict's silver lining, and it ties back to the main goal of this book: achieving a vivid, brilliantly lived life.

When the pain and suffering of conflict disappear, what we can grow into is even greater beauty—in this life and beyond.

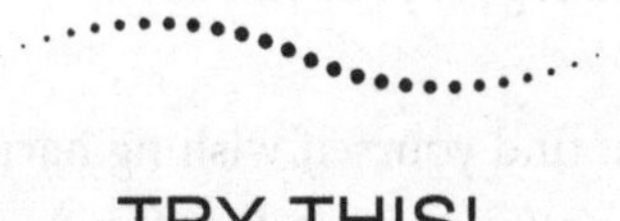

TRY THIS!

Think back to a recent time when you experienced conflict. Visualize yourself as you were responding to the other person just moments before you felt conflicted. Consider your body language, voice, mind-set, and any emotions you were feeling. Then visualize how you responded to any aggressive energy you might have felt coming from the other person and from yourself. Did you become irrational? Why? Finally, consider various energy tools you can draw from to get harmonized and flowing if this specific conflicting situation comes up again.

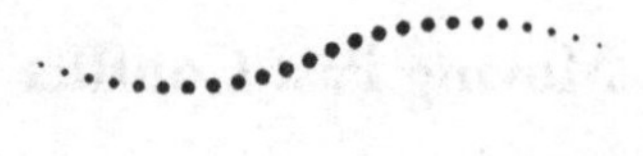

Exercises and Practices

1. An end-of-the-day practice visualization: Imagine a circumstance in which you experienced conflict. Visualize yourself in the situation; bring as many senses into play as you can. Using your mind's eye to freeze the action at a variety of different points, ask yourself what you could have done to turn off what was triggering conflict in you, and what you could have turned on to achieve balance and peaceful resolution. Apply these lessons the next time you are in a similar situation.

2. The next time you feel conflict with another individual, take a breath. Focus on resolving the conflict rather than being right. Remember, most of what is being said may or may not be true, so the conflict—which is draining you—may not even be worth it. Sometimes things don't matter in terms of who is right or wrong. Let yourself radiate in Virtue instead, and regain your flow.

3. The next time you find yourself wishing harm or ill feelings toward someone, tell yourself immediately: *My mind is attached. This is not my true Self.* Then step back, and put your mind back into flow. If you cannot, focus on one or more universal Virtues. Listen closely and well. Wait for a window of virtuous response to open, and then respond fluidly and gently, letting the bright energy of your true Self and original nature radiate forward.

4. Work with swarming energy to help manage conflict. Put together a set of tools including sound, music, and art that function to help you establish balance before and after conflicts pop up in your daily life. I always encourage using your cell phone or other electronic device to file these. Remember combinations of sounds, colors, visuals, and language amplify the effect.

5. Put on a piece of calming music or natural sound that is ideally twelve minutes in length, and meditate. In a seated position, calm and center yourself. Imagine how relaxed you feel right before a great night's sleep. Scan your body to feel all your muscles becoming less tense and softening. Feel your mind unknotting. As you do so, concentrate on your breathing, and imagine good energy streaming into you as you breathe in. As you breathe out, release any conflicting emotions you've been holding inside. With your hand over your heart, acknowledge the earth and the Universe for its restorative and protective energy. Send it your love. Feel its love flowing through you.

8

USING ENERGY TO REVERSE DETRIMENTAL AGGRESSION

Aggression, like every other part of human behavior
we take for granted, is a challenging engineering problem!

—Steven Pinker

Most of us have encountered individuals who have aggressively over-reacted. Perhaps it was a driver who was tailgating you and lost his cool, nearly causing an accident. Or maybe it was a salesperson who tried to sell you a certain product. Or perhaps it was someone you met at a social occasion who was "all over" everyone. Or perhaps your own aggression has made you uncomfortable at times or sent you into detrimental behaviors.

When we think of aggression, we usually define the term as something negative. Yet all aggression is certainly not bad. It is a natural, normal, and healthy human emotion. As we previously discussed, it can be the driving force behind much goodness, creativity, discovery, and success. But aggression's flipside—its harmful drive—needs to be channeled positively or made to cease (when channeling positively is not possible), or it can fly out of control. Take, for example, an individual who is angry that he wasn't hired for a job he really wanted. He can rechannel this emotion and the energy it provides into something positive and constructive. For him, this may mean taking a close look at his resumé and other documents he prepared for this prospective employer, figuring out what improvements he can make so that he presents as a stronger candidate—and then taking action to make these improvements. He may also rechannel some of his energy into identifying a list of other potential and ideal employers to which he can apply. When our aggressions do get out of control, they inhibit performance, block access to higher quality energy, and steer attention into areas that can cause further problems.

Essentially, there are two forms of aggression: destructive aggressive energy and constructive aggressive energy. When we are operating at our best, we nurture aggression's constructive energies and regulate its harmful ones. The challenge is to identify your aggressions as you feel them, and to recognize them as being constructive or damaging. Then you must regulate them by making them cease, channeling them positively (when destructive), or funneling them (when constructive) into beneficial directions, such as fueling creative solutions, getting out of gridlock, or simply getting a job done.

The key to dealing with aggression is not ignoring it. Ignoring your aggression won't get rid of its harmful twists and turns. Nor will it give you the opportunity to capitalize on and use it to fuel positive endeavors. By not confronting it, the aggression you feel will start coming out "sideways" in other situations; for example, a person who is angry at his boss ignores it and then engages in road rage on his drive home.

Unattended aggression also presents a long list of personal health concerns, including fatigue, heart attack, stroke, headaches, and sleeplessness. The good news is that each of these symptoms offers you a window of opportunity to make positive adjustments in your energy, so be sure to pay attention to them.

Compensating to Regulate

Our ability to compensate for things that we expect to happen is known as *behavioral tolerance.* Compensation is part of your response to listening to your body-mind-spirit, and is a great tool toward achieving better and balanced performance in whatever you do. Furthermore, it can help you regulate feelings of aggression in your life.

For a simple example of how the mind uses compensation, let's consider the negative effects of alcohol on driving. Knowing how alcohol will impair you, your mind can try to compensate by attempting to regulate your actions. However, in order to do this, your brain needs to be familiar with the effects of alcohol. If you've never had a sip of alcohol in your life and don't have a sense of what impairments to expect, your brain won't know how to balance out your actions to compensate. This is why blood-alcohol contents are somewhat debatable. A person who does not use alcohol regularly would be a danger after consuming much less than someone who has several drinks every day.

Another part of compensation has to do with your ability to experience what you expect. This is the principle behind the placebo effect. Countless studies have been conducted in which one group of test subjects is given a drug, while a control group is given an inactive sugar pill. Both groups are told they have received the true medication and what it is expected to achieve. While those who received the drug will experience its effects, those in the control group will often experience the same effects simply because they expect to. The takeaway point from this test is that the mind is able to compensate for certain energies that affect it, based on previous experience and expectations.

Practicing compensation—by being mindful of the peripheral signs of your aggression and adjusting—makes a significant difference in your ability to self-regulate in general and in feelings of aggression. So if you are feeling aggressive, make yourself aware of the peripheral signs that arise inside you. This will help you catch potentially destructive aggression sooner—before it becomes a problem—and give you choice as to how you want to proceed. It will also help you use your positive aggressive energy reasonably and constructively.

On-the-Spot Fixes

Sometimes you have to attend to feelings of negative aggression on the fly. This usually calls for immediate adjustment, and it differs from introspecting to decide whether you think operating this way is to your advantage (mentally, physically, and spiritually) or not.

When you are on the fly, you will notice that there is a distinct feeling to the spectrum of time from when you have "almost" entered into an aggressive mind-set to when that mind-set is chronic. I am suggesting that you learn to feel into this window of time and energy. Learn to identify the window, especially on the fly. The advantage to recognizing this "almost" stage of negative aggression is that you can learn to compensate for it and then get yourself back to a balanced mind-set energetically.

When you feel you have entered this zone of "almost" aggressive mind, start compensating by telling yourself firmly that you need to disengage from it. Say to yourself, *This is negative energy*, and then pause; wait before you do anything else. Just make yourself aware until the best window for a good response—one rooted in your true nature—opens.

Patience is the antidote to negative aggression. Take a nice slow breath, and tell yourself that the feeling will pass. When it does, you will be better able to respond to the specific life situation you are in.

In the meantime, you can compensate by emptying and calming your mind, bringing your full awareness to the situation. Further compensate by putting on your most neutral facial expression—or even better, a kind, tolerant, and compassionate facial expression. Feel into the energy of Virtue, which connects you to your highest-level energy resources of pure Self. In this way, you will be acting from the vantage point of who you are at your truest.

This is also a good time in the process to call to mind any visualization, *power words*, or musical memory you have practiced that can bring immediate, positive, and calming energy. As you do so, let that good energy flow through your mind and body. Use this exercise to give you the informed power you need to regulate your aggression and to mindfully generate your best, most authentic response. As has been mentioned before, the more you have used your chosen visualization in the past, the better it will work in instances when you truly need it—and need it quickly.

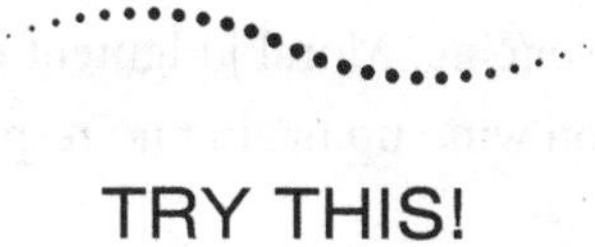

TRY THIS!

Next time you enter the "almost" zone of negative aggression, practice compensation by telling yourself this is negative energy. Take a slow breath and don't do anything. Detach from the persona functioning on this energy. Tell yourself, *This is not who I really am or want to be. This is not the energy—the informed power—of my original nature, which is guided by Virtue, the Universal Principle of yin-yang, and Self.* Feel into the negative energy (but not too long); identify it as bad for you; and redirect it to flow through you without inciting additional thoughts, feelings, or actions. Rebalance your mind with a visual or sound you have stored in your memory for times like this. Mindfully listen. Respond to the situation that triggered your aggressive response when the best opportunity arises.

Increase Activities that Boost Moral Judgment

From the perspective of mind-body medicine, cultivating the subtler and higher quality energy of higher moral judgment regulates and manages harmful aggressive and antisocial behaviors that your mind has attached to. We have discussed positive aggression as a way to drive goals you wish to pursue. But in order to self-regulate proficiently, you need to be mindful of the moral judgment that is (or is not) weighing in on—and is part of the basis for—your decisions and their outcomes.

At its most general level, moral judgment is your basis for identifying right and wrong. It is the interaction of the data that is before you—what you observe or experience (even if that is a private aspiration, thought, or feeling)—with what you value, and how that then shapes your opinions on what you are experiencing. Moral judgment ultimately impacts how you respond, even if you wind up having no response.

Here is how it works:

1. You experience something.
2. Your mind fetches a value that you have stored in memory.
3. This value helps you formulate an opinion.
4. You respond (or not).

What makes this a little tricky is that you can go from observation to response in milliseconds. If you have no value weighing in on what you are witnessing, you will have no opinion—and therefore, no response. The greater the value, the stronger your opinion, and the more intense your response.

Consider an individual who is part of a business team for an organization. On this particular day, the entire team has been assigned to what he sees as menial work. He values doing only higher-level work, such as forecasting product trends for the organization. Even though the menial work he has been asked to do is not outside his job description and will last only one day, his opinion of it is one of disapproval. He judges this activity as "below him." As a result, he becomes unhappy and starts showing attitude to his fellow teammates, as well as his supervisor. He later recognizes that his actions have added tension to his relationships at work and now regrets having lost control. This added strain is now a drain on his energies.

Being mindful, and acting more in sync with his original nature and Universal Virtue (honesty, compassion, acceptance, peace, and unconditional love) would have given him the informed power to self-regulate his behaviors so they turned out more in line with his best interests.

Being mindful, and acting more in sync with his original nature and Universal Virtue would have also created a window to rechannel his aggression. By rechanneling his harmful aggressions, he could have used them to personally motivate a search for more meaningful and satisfying employment. To do any of this, however, he needs to involve himself in activities that boost the quality of his moral judgment—activities that better explore and understand his basis for tagging something right (okay) or wrong (not okay) for him and others.

Increasing activities to boost moral judgment is especially important since distractions are numerous and life seems to get busier all the time—not to mention our growing reliance on electronics that often keep us focused superficially. We too easily allow much of our time to be used spending and cultivating the lower level energies, which leaves us drained. And so much of this is the result of habit (old dysfunctional procedures). I am not saying such activities should be avoided; what I am saying is that they need to be balanced with high-quality, energy-cultivating activities.

From the perspective of Western medicine, Dr. Mario F. Mendez wrote in the *CNS Spectrums* journal that "morality may be innate to the human brain."[1] Within this view, the practice of Virtue is consistent with generating behaviors that harmonize survival with other individuals and enhance our appreciation of their own thinking, opinions, and feelings.

One individual I was working with a short while ago told me that she used to go home after work, have dinner with her family (sometimes a sit-down meal though not always), have dessert, and then head to the bedroom to watch what she referred to as mindless shows—anything to take her mind off of the day's stressors. Weekends were similar, except that rather than working, she and her husband and three boys were out and about all day, both Saturday and Sunday, taking classes, shopping, traveling to relatives', and participating in mostly light conversation—nothing too heavy—but sometimes financial and business talk. She and her husband saw their job as keeping the kids busy—"keeps them out of trouble," she said. She had a point about the children; they were learning some nice skills in addition to what they learned in school. But the constant busyness energetically drained them all. Starting their next week at an energy deficit only added to their individual and family stress throughout the week.

They needed to set aside more time during weekdays and weekends for higher-quality energy cultivation at all levels, but especially the higher, subtler energies—which, when unblocked and accessible, would give her and her family the restoration and fuel for their many activities. This energy helps build positive aggression and staves off negative.

Although the mindless television programming could potentially plug some energy drain, the shows did little to restore and cultivate the necessary higher quality energy, because the information and power they transferred was not nurturing her deeper Self. So at best, restoration was incomplete; and at worst, it helped create new circuits (templates) for behaviors that were impractical or harmful to their best interests.

In contrast, meditation, visualization, reflection, tai chi, yoga, chi kung—all contribute to higher energy gains. Any of these can function as a reasonable substitute. But there is another source for cultivating subtler, higher quality energy that will transfer and transform into the daily energy you need to generate healthy aggressions and avoid detrimental ones. It is the informed power of moral judgment, it is related to the cultivation of Virtue, and it is available in all of the arts, sciences, and spiritual texts. This energy restores and nurtures all three levels of consciousness of spirit, mind, and body. In mind-body medicine, we believe moral judgment is powerful enough to establish pathways for new procedures in the mind and, hence, new circuits in your brain.

Iconic author and philosopher John Gardner once said that societies live and die by the virtue within the fictions they believe.[2] He was referring to the existence and presentation of values in creative writings. You can, however, substitute any art's values within his model, and it will still have the same effect.

We have already talked about the energetic power of syncing with Universal Virtue in order to reboot your original nature. I now want to suggest that by exploring the values, ethical content, and decision-making reasoning that you can find in your favorite art(s), you can boost your own ethical energy, and more solidly and energetically sync to the power of Universal Virtue. This will open up your full energy flow, maximize your overall performance, and strengthen your mind at all levels.

When a person's moral judgment is left uncultivated, mostly unexplored, or explored at superficial levels, it can result in that individual's attachment to harmful aggressive energy for several reasons. The lack of information with which to strongly and convincingly reason things out, as well as to empathize morally and respond appropriately helps generate the situations that are not in your best interests and could be dangerous to you and others. They can roll over into low self-confidence and shaky involvements, with less trust in self and in others. All of this brings more stress, anxiety, depression, and immunity-related illness into one's life.

On the other hand, activities that will charge your creative mind and help you develop a deeper sense of morality can cultivate the high quality and abundant energy you need to restore balance and flow into your life. These activities are often what we associate with right-brain undertakings and can be the source of a lot of entertainment and fun.

You can, for example, tap into arts like film, literature, poetry, and music; read philosophical and spiritual texts; or participate in philosophical and spiritual conversations to connect with these energies. Combined with visualization, reflection, and meditation, you create new pathways (circuits) to better thinking, feeling, and performing. Each of these activities, in turn, generates a cycle of energy and reward that will strengthen your mind with greater moral reasoning, personal procedures for getting things done and for solving skills, a more satisfying worldview, and heightened spirituality. Together, they will generate a high-quality swarmed energy and a powerful, flowing, and informed mind.

Make the Time for Moral Cultivation

All of this exploration into moral judgment may sound like a luxury. You may say that you do not have the time for such artistic/intellectual appreciation. But I would like to gently suggest that, energetically speaking, this component of your total energy cultivation is necessary. You need to make the time for such activities because they not only help you refresh to your original nature that is aligned to Universal Values, but they restore your psychic and physical energy as well. You cannot expect your body and mind to push the pedal to the metal 24/7 without restoration. And that means more than just plugging your energy drains. Increasing your moral energy makes you more sensitive to energies that are good for you (and for others) and helps you build a feedback loop with them. Once your moral reasoning gets involved—those areas of your brain that are affected by *serotonin* and dopamine—you feel virtuous, happy, and rewarded. You begin to prefer thinking and acting this way.

Your perceptions, feelings, motivations, and rewards all synchronize into a positive and stronger energy loop. And this momentum of high, well-informed power (positive aggression) allows you to create stronger procedures to function with less effort—pursuing those things each day that require and burn your energy, and replenishing yourself with high quality energy to keep you flowing. It is your job, however, to involve your thinking, higher level brain, learning from and exploring moral cultivation more deeply, and seeking the reward of making better life choices to achieve optimum-level performance.

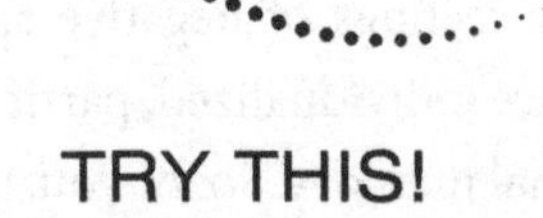

TRY THIS!

This activity works well solo or with others. Choose any piece of art that you like. It can be a story, quality film, and so on. Then examine what overall human action is presented within (and by) the composition.

Identify what opinion the artist wants you to formulate of the human action presented in the piece. Consider if the composer wants you to agree or to disagree with such action. (This is different from what your personal opinion of the action is.) Also consider how emotive an opinion the composer is attempting to elicit, and feel the energy of this opinion.

Now identify the "value" significance of the presented action in light of the opinion the composer is trying to develop in you. Does the composer want you to see the value of love, loyalty, friendship, family, solitude? Consider whether this value might have the potential to lead you to higher-quality good in your life, and if so, how it can accomplish that. Think about action steps you may need to take to activate this value. Think of several ways to perpetrate it in your own life right away and long term. How can you use it to positively affect the lives of others?

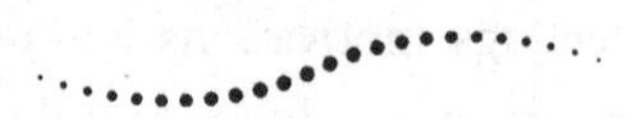

Using Scent to Achieve Balance

The quickest brain fix is scent. This is because it will bypasss your thinking brain and go right to where things can transform in seconds or less. If you have already used scent during certain meditations and visualizations, it will pay off here. If not, this is a great time to start.

Lavender, cedar, sandalwood, chamomile, lemon, and vanilla have been known to reduce feelings of negative aggression and stress. But many aspects of scent are individualized, particularly when you combine fragrance with emotional memory. So for you, the scent of beach oils and sunscreens may work as an aggression buster; for someone else, it may pump them up if they attach the scent to athletics like seaside volleyball, sailing, or fishing.

Start now with scents that you think may work; but keep in mind that you can create your own *armamentarium* by using fragrances and oils during emotionally pleasant times as well—when you feel balanced and beautiful. The idea is to experiment, have fun, and use your imagination as you continue to look for new fragrances that vaporize negative aggression from you. Be sure to ingrain these moments and scents into your memory so that you can pull them out when necessary and use them to combat these negative feelings.

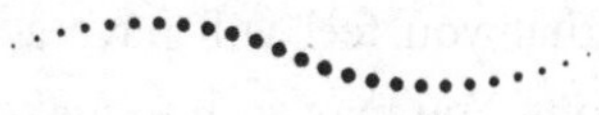

TRY THIS!

Find a fragrance that calms you down. Use it in calm moments and when you want to enhance relaxation. (Perfumes, colognes, and oils all work.) Use it often, applying it whenever you need or anticipate needing a little extra calming energy throughout your day.

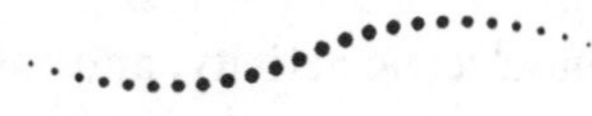

Using Color to Calm

Color also works to reverse harmful aggression. Green is effective in this, as are blue and white. You may have a picture with greens or blues or glistening whites that is already ingrained in your memory. If so, use that one, but if not, find one. Remember, the more you enjoy the photo or artwork and anticipate its calming effects, the better it will work.

It is also a good idea to remain sensitive to colors in nature and in your other environments. Feel into their energy. Invite their energy into you and feel their specific empowering characteristics, as well as how they inform you. This will lead you to find new colors that can help to guide you away from negative aggressions.

Music and Natural Sound

Just as they moderate other emotions, songs and natural sounds offer a nice way to alleviate negative aggressions as you experience them and even beforehand, when you anticipate them. The musical concepts to reverse anxiety that were presented previously will apply here as well;

simply choose songs that you feel will have a tranquilizing effect on your negative aggressions. You may wish to make more than one playlist to refer to more than one type of negatively aggressive behavior—e.g., workplace, athletics, and relationships.

Using Language

I love the magnificence of linguistic energy and all you can do with it. It is amazing that you can take a single word like "honesty," for instance, and focus on it in a meditation, transferring and transforming its subtle energy into the body's bioelectric activity; and then into action, feeling, more thought, and memory—for future use—via your body-mind-spirit connection. The informed power of language is enormous, and you can even use it as a way to transfer energy to others.

Let's take a look at how you can use language for the early detection of harmful aggression and how language can help rechannel that aggression into more functional energy.

Going back for a moment to the notion of intentionally inhibiting a word, expression, thought, idea, or action, remember that the more you inhibit it, the more difficult it becomes to engage. So the idea is to first identify language that makes you susceptible to certain aggressions—e.g., when you say (or think) thus and thus, you often land in a heated argument with your partner or another specific individual in your life. This language can take many forms for many people, but it commonly includes harsh words; emotionally cold language (especially where warmer, more sensitive language is more appropriate); and words that deal with a certain subject, person, or place. Once you identify this language, you can use it to cue you that you are about to enter into an aggressive mind-set.

In order to help you identify such language, try reflecting on times when you became aggressive. Again, you will be paying attention to the spectrum of feeling so that you can begin to identify language that appears in the "almost" category—before you become fully aggressive. Note, too, if you feel the absence of language or "stuck for words." Once you are aware of such cues, you are in a window of opportunity to turn off your rising aggressive energies before they become damaging. Disengaging these triggers inhibits them from driving the specific aggressions they are attached to the next time you are in this or a similar situation. By being mindful of when you enter this stage, you can intervene, rechannel the rising aggression, or prevent it altogether.

Next, use your visualization to attach positive language that will prompt and foster appropriate and advantageous thinking, feeling, and behaving within the situation. Visualize yourself acting and thinking out of honesty, compassion, acceptance, tolerance, peace, and love in the moment. By adding this language to your visualization at strategic points in the narrative, you help it kick in, powering up and guiding you to an optimized, real-time performance.

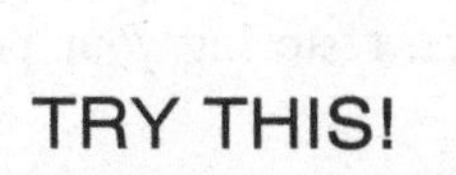

TRY THIS!

The next time you experience feelings of aggression, stop them and step back from the situation. Take a time out to think and reflect. Ask yourself about what is making you aggressive, and consider whether or not that feeling is appropriate to the situation at hand. Think about both your goal in this situation and what others are looking to achieve. Ask yourself if you are responding from a dysfunctional belief system, and reflect on what happened the last time you responded this way.

Once you have considered all of this, take charge and determine which thoughts, feelings, and actions you want to activate and which ones you want to inhibit. After you know which energies you want to inhibit, tell yourself firmly that these are negative energies. Listen to yourself, and respond with your best sensibility.

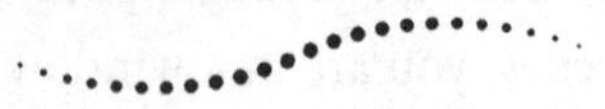

Other Ways to Deal with Negative Aggression

In addition to what we've already covered, there are several other ways that you can constructively deal with aggression.

For example, you can use humor to help dissolve it. This can work at home, at work, and in your relationships. However, there is a word of caution here: take care not to go too far. Sometimes people use teasing, for example, to ease aggressions. But joking around can make other people anxious and frustrated. So you need to be careful, as such feelings can spread quickly.

Another way to deal with harmful aggressive energies is through your family, organizational, and social cultures. Celebrations, dinners, sporting events, as well as arts and spiritual events offer ways to relieve aggressions and rebalance, restoring your positive energy and getting you back in the saddle.

A third way to deal with aggression is to spend time in nature. Oftentimes, all you need is a brief walk outside to let go of negative aggressions and set your mind's restart button. If you don't have time for a walk, try glancing out the window. Put a smile on your face as you do, taking advantage of those free feel-good hormones via the increased light rays (they shift your blood chemistry from irritated to happy). Choose to flow with the goodness and positivity of the energy you see and encounter. Don't let negative aggressions charge the rest of your day with their dysfunction; transfer and transform higher quality energy throughout your entire being and change the course of your day. Then you can pass that higher quality energy forward.

Cultivating Positive Aggressive Energy

As was briefly discussed earlier, aggression is not inherently bad. In fact, it can provide that extra power and energy we need to accomplish a goal. As such, there are situations in which you want to cultivate aggression functionally in order to optimize performance and judgment.

For example, aggression can be used as a motivator. Disengagement and lack of interest takes its toll in many life situations we'd like to improve. Here, the brain issues just enough of the right dose of its aggression-related hormones (adrenaline, cortisol, testosterone) to help you optimize your talents to get the job done. For the individual who has had difficulty getting a new exercise program or an academic, business, or artistic pursuit off the ground, getting angry with the status quo may be just the thing. But in order to do this, you have to put yourself into a positive mind-set and allow yourself to think constructively—to see and establish the solution.

Aggressive energy can also be used to identify and adjust unreasonable demands on your lifestyle with peaceful solutions. For instance, an individual I know very successfully rechanneled the potentially damaging influence of envy he'd felt for friends who had graduated high school with him and had already completed graduate school; this motivated his own pursuit of higher education and brought him more satisfaction and peace in life.

Another situation in which aggressive energy can be useful is when you need help sharing or exploring important information that is otherwise difficult for you. Another individual I know had his identity stolen recently, and he harbored very aggressive feelings as a result of the incident. Rechanneling this energy, he cut through a myriad of bureaucratic obstacles and explored the possibilities of the theft so expeditiously that all stolen monies were retrieved and any further damages stopped.

Finally, aggression (competitive or otherwise) can be used to get creative. Use what's stirring you up to explore and flow deeper into a situation.

Obviously, something has your attention. This could be anything from coming up with new football-game strategies to designing innovative choreography for modern dance to writing an article or poem. All of these creative endeavors can be driven, heightened, and kept flowing by funneling your aggressive energy toward their creative exploration.

Each of these requires rechanneling the energy of aggression into a positive direction. Make the practices of mindfulness and calmness primary in your life so you can sustain an alert yet calm and focused mind-set. Regular practice will make this a prominent mind-set for you over time.

Exercises and Practices

1. The next time you are feeling the stress of overaggressiveness, try a massage. Good for keeping your aggressions in check, massage is known to increase your levels of feel-good hormones (serotonin, dopamine) and balance levels of fight-or-flight chemicals (adrenaline, cortisol) to keep appropriate levels in your blood.

2. Make a special playlist of songs designed to vaporize any harmful aggressions.

3. Exercise daily (and especially when feeling in an aggressive zone). Exercise is capable of balancing your serotonin levels and increasing endorphins, helping you to ward off harmful aggressions, and replace feelings of ill-ease and malaise with a cascade of feel-good chemistry that may be just enough to shift your focus and mind-set.

4. Use the informed power of happy memories to reverse aggressive feelings.

9

USING ENERGY TO BEAT OBSESSION

The new physics provides a modern version
of ancient spirituality. In a universe made out of energy,
everything is entangled; everything is one.

—BRUCE LIPTON

Obsessions . . . they are so common and they come in many packages. Some people obsess over tiny problems. Others obsess over larger things that could happen to them even though these things have a history of never coming to fruition. Every day, intrusive thoughts can enter your mind and disturb your tranquility. Sometimes, they veer us off course and we can't get rid of them. You can receive ninety compliments and one criticism, yet you keep going over the single criticism in your head. Then there is that proverbial incident that happened long ago that you just can't let go of—it comes up in your mind like clockwork; all it takes is the slightest trigger. You wonder: *What's up with that; why do I keep caring about this incident?* Your mind's repeat button gets stuck on a thought, story, or picture. Then it plays it over and over in your head. The problem is that we are all vulnerable to these kinds of looping thoughts, and having a caring nature means we may perseverate on a situation we cannot control. But these invasive circles of thinking can mess up your current endeavors and plans.

The Informed Power of Nonstop Negative Thinking

Sometimes you can get stuck on what feels like a nonstop wheel of negative thinking. This trek is often linked to incidents from your past, such as something you revealed about yourself to a coworker a day ago or a rude comment someone you had a crush on may have made to you years ago.

There are many reasons why our minds attach to such things. Some are much easier to identify and deal with than others, as there may be multiple layers of causes that you may or may not be conscious of. Some causes may have even occurred while you were still in your mother's womb, while others are rooted in your life experiences; and others are from both. Nonetheless, at one time or another, most of us feel some form of worrisome thinking that we go around and around on, with no apparent end or solution in sight.

It is perfectly natural to think your worries are over in an attempt to get a grip on them and find solutions. However, they may get the best of you and start playing like a nonstop movie in your mind. Then, they can energetically turn into a troublesome emotional cycle of depression, grief, envy, or anger. This cycle of thought and feeling is called *rumination*. Unfortunately, it doesn't stop there.

Your mind likes attaching itself to similar content, so you are likely to attach to other life issues that levy similar emotional arousal. This, in part, explains why, when you are feeling great, you tend to ride on waves of happiness, and when you are feeling sad, you tend to dive into more distress. It also means that when you are angry, you very quickly—and without much warning—attach to your favorite half dozen or so things that peeve you. Instead of being upset over one thing, now your favorite irritations are orbiting your mind and pushing buttons. Next thing you know, they are firing all kinds of patterns across your mind and throughout your body—which are not in your best interests mentally or physically.

This energetic tendency of attaching to like emotional content is known as *emotional congruency*. When you are feeling good, this energy pattern sends you on a pleasure-seeking mission for more reward. This can, however, quickly stress you out and wreak havoc on your focus, contributing to a slippery slope of addictive or risky behaviors, such as overworking, overeating, or even overexercising. All of these drain your energy, do nothing to replace it, and develop into automatic behaviors that can run under your radar and be further problematic.

One individual I know involved himself in the same risky behavior in reaction to both good or bad news. His habit was to drive his sports car at very high speeds—and it didn't matter if he was alone in his car or with friends. You could see the "procedure" kicking in as if a potentially harmful chemical had been released in his bloodstream and a current of electricity had just been turned on in his brain. In fact, they had.

In holistic medicine, we believe such attachment lowers quality energy patterns and is damaging to short- and long-term performance. It weakens the mind and body, and blocks the spirit. It takes you out of your element, disenfranchises you from your higher Self and its nurturing energy, disengages your mindfulness, and misdirects you during important moments. This negatively impacts your decision making, overall performance, and self-confidence in respect to future endeavors. We see this interruption in flow as something that needs to be addressed and changed.

Remember, everyone experiences such moments to some extent; it's how you respond that matters. As such, from the perspective of holistic medicine, we also view these moments as great opportunities to strengthen and cultivate the mind. This cultivation carries its own loops of thought, feeling, procedures, and feel-good energy—the kind of feedback you want so you can keep flowing. So how do you get there?

Plug Your Energy Drain

Your first job is to get out of the obsession trap and plug the energy drain. One way to start reversing the power of obsession and working toward balance is to identify—again, early in the spectrum—when you feel caught (or about to get stuck) in this kind of unproductive, consuming energy rut.

Once you have identified that you have an obsession, take a step back and work to plug the drain. You can initially do this by energetically feeling into the emotion and telling yourself this is not you—this is not the energy of your true Self; this is an energy trap. Tell yourself things are probably not as bad as you think; that you will let this caustic energy flow through you, and you will not let it back in.

After you have gotten rid of all of the bad energy, you need to seal the drain so that the plug doesn't break free. There are several ways you can do this.

Psychologically, distraction helps. This is why a coach's whistle works to shift an athlete's attention, and why some elementary school teachers and parents (by habit or by strategy) clap their hands loudly to quickly move a child from one behavior to another. This is the time to take out one of your "toys," such as a new piece of exercise or musical equipment, and use it to take your mind off its destructive course—to put it on something that makes you happy.

Another thing you can do to stop the energy pattern of obsessions from draining you is to set a time limit for yourself. Tell yourself, *I will think about this concern for fifteen minutes and fifteen minutes only. Then I will get on to the task at hand.*

Or take a break and tell yourself that you will give your concern more time and better-quality thought later, such as after lunch or following your afternoon meeting. Or you might want to wait even longer, telling yourself that you will wait till the next weekend to think things through—so that you can approach the concern with fresh perspective and more positive energy. This tactic frees you up momentarily, helps set a different energy pattern, and gives you the additional mental strength you need to take a look at things later.

You can also help seal the drain by involving yourself in feel-good, energy-building activities. Keep these simple, and don't take on too much. Feel into whatever activity you choose. If it is a rhythmic activity like sweeping a floor, feel into the rhythm. If it is rooting like working with your hands in a garden, feel into the rootedness. Do something small and positive, and let its energy refresh you.

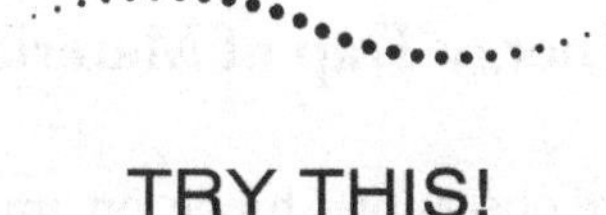

TRY THIS!

Try this meditation outdoors; if you can't get out, do it indoors via a picture slideshow.

Start by taking your shoes off and walking barefoot on the grass. Feel the cool moisture travel straight through the bottom of your feet. Feel your body absorb energy up from the earth. Visualize this energy as a warm, nourishing, vibrant green.

Imagine this energy circulating within you. Imagine it flowing up over the crown of your head, down your back, and down into the earth again, in a circular motion. As it flows, imagine it cleansing you of toxic feelings that may be weighing you down physically and mentally. Direct these negative energies into the earth—imagine them flowing into the earth. The earth can handle these poisons, you cannot.

Repeat this activity for as long as you are comfortable, and do it often. Feel your mind clearing and loosening each time you draw in more energy. Breathe the entire image into your body deeply and slowly—in through your nose and exhaled through your mouth. Look around your environment or an imagined favorite one.

Now, close your eyes and turn the picture green; breathe it all in. Imagine this cleansing energy rising through your limbs, through muscle and bone, to your heart. Feel its rising energy flowing through you. Let it purify and warm your heart. As you exhale, feel into and visualize the energy of your dreams flowing outward in peace and joy. Feel the calm exhilaration of consciously participating in this energy. Use this meditation to revitalize often.

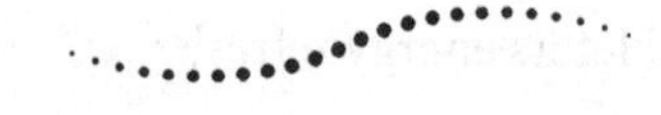

The Energy Trap of Materialism

Although many of our obsessions hinge on immaterial things, such as actions we took or words we said (or need to do or say), it is also important to be aware of obsessing about material possessions you don't need. Once you send your mind the message through the repetitions of thought, feeling, or action that unnecessary material things should be pursued, it will automatically drive your focus to these pursuits, spending more and more of your energy trying to acquire them for you. This will not only steer you off course, generating low-quality satisfaction in life, but it will also block your higher-quality energy resources of mind-spirit while constantly draining your lower energies. This will catch you in a tailspin of negative energy returns, which then creates further problems—cognitively, emotionally, physically, and spiritually. Unable to replenish your energy, your mind is programming itself to keep its constant focus on only energy-draining concerns. So the question becomes, How do you unblock it and get it on a healthier track?

You can do this by connecting with your highest mind—your spiritual mind. Because the nature of this mind is spiritual, it will not be attracted to the material/physical world pursuits that are lowering your energy and keeping you there. Your spiritual mind will instead be attracted to higher spiritual energy in the form of balance and Virtue; and it will seek to cultivate this energy in your daily endeavors, refreshing and replenishing your energy supply for daily functions.

Through meditation, you can reopen your tri-level consciousness and feel into the energy and dreams of your spiritual mind. As you do, you will discover they easily articulate as feelings, for they are associated with the energy of Virtue—honesty, compassion, acceptance, peace, and unconditional love—and with balance. If you increase your concentration in this mind-set, you will be able to see where the energies of Virtue and complementarity (yin-yang) can be applied and evolved into various aspects of your life. This will help to restore your full-being consciousness and access to its higher quality energy. It will help you limit physical and mental energy drains, and place you in a healthier cycle of purpose, joy, and energy cultivation.

Why Am I So Hung Up On . . . ?

When you look at the bigger picture, you can sometimes see a specific stressor that is making you obsess. Finding this stressor can free your mind from obsessing and energy loss. Some people, for example, get trapped in an ongoing habit of getting fixated and anxious every time they have to be somewhere on time—so much so that it is a predictable response whenever they are in a situation where punctuality is concerned. As they try to get to their commitment on time, they become more and more stressed and fixated on peripheral things, such as finding their jogging sneakers, which aren't where they last put them, or finding an article of clothing they want to wear, or returning an inconsequential phone call to a family member. None of these concerns has anything to do with their current commitment, but their fixation makes them feel like they have no choice but to follow their diversion—as if they are being pulled by a magnet. And in a way, they are.

Such traps are completely unrelated to making it to a commitment on time, functioning as diversions to some larger concern that is going on in the unconscious mind. What's more, one's focus can get hung up in just seconds. It seems to people caught in these obsessions that no matter what they do—e.g., set an alarm or timer—they get hooked; and if it is not one thing that's diverted their focus, it's another. This kind of ongoing obsession can be the source of much anxiety and even misery for individuals until they identify the pattern and its root.

One person I know found herself in this pattern of being chronically late. With introspection, she discovered that her fixation on unrelated tasks and items was linked to her participation in activities that she did not want to be doing. Once she identified the pattern, she was able to change commitments to activities more nurturing to her Self.

Many of us get trapped in similar patterns. We wonder what is wrong with us and why we are so hung up over something that has apparently nothing to do with the matters at hand. Such obsessions are more common than you may think. Once you have identified the patterns, however, you have the opportunity to shed them and aim yourself in a much more satisfying direction.

What You Can Do

One way to deal with this kind of obsessing is to make yourself aware of what other issues (in the bigger picture) may be adding stress to your behavior, and identify your predictable responses to those—e.g., *When I am pressed for time, I feel stressed, and that often makes me focus on unrelated things—like sneakers or unconnected conversation.* Look for the patterns; they will reveal how you get trapped. Then look for ways to relieve them.

Some circumstances are easier to deal with than others. For example, if your stressor is that you are rushed; giving yourself more preparation time might alleviate your stress and its subsequent obsessions, and plug your energy drain. But it's not always that simple.

Many stressors are layered like this. For instance, no matter how early you start trying to get into motion, it sometimes won't eliminate nerve-wracking, last-minute obsessions from piling up. This may be your cue to look deeper into what's going on.

Consider the following example: Kate Larson is a VP for an advertising firm. She is relatively new at the job and has been burning the midnight oil working on projects for clients. When she finally gets to bed, she has a hard time getting to sleep and wakes up a few times before morning. She is also having a hard time getting back to sleep. Lately, she has been obsessing over several things—her health, which is primarily good, but also things that could go wrong in her house, such as leaving doors unlocked or the water running. She also can't stop thinking about the quality of her work lately.

In an effort to get to the root of the problem, Kate tries some introspection. First, she is able to see that the things she obsesses on are things she usually obsesses on. She thinks of times when her mind feels freer and asks herself what changes. This helps illuminate a pattern that traps her into obsessing. The pattern, she takes note, is sparked by her lack of good-quality sleep, then the onset of insomnia. Once she is unable to sleep, she begins to ruminate about current work projects, which then spreads to obsessions over unlocked doors, left-on stoves, and health issues.

So one of Kate's potential energy traps is her unhealthy sleep habit. Digging deeper, she sees another potential energy trap: her preference to shield herself from having to confront clients with more reasonable schedules than the ones they have proposed to her, and the necessary aggression she needs to confront them.

Although everyone's patterns may be different, what's similar is the need to dig in and take a look at what your energy looks and feels like when you are on top of your game, and what it looks like when you are obsessing or ruminating. Start here. Ask yourself what has changed. Use that as a starting point for locating the energy that traps you into your own circular thinking and behavior.

Listen to Your Self

In order to accurately identify things that change in you from when you're feeling on top of your game to feeling totally drained, you need to practice listening to your Self. This practice is a core element of this book. It allows you to function at your energetic optimum, supplying you with the right energy (juice and information) for specific tasks.

As you practice listening to your Self, I want to gently suggest that you do so with honesty, compassion, acceptance, peace, and unconditional love. Again, feel into the energy of Universal Virtue and let it flow through you, empowering and informing you. In combination with the principle of yin-yang, this high quality energy will guide you beyond the level of conditioned desires—which are the wants of others, the media, and your culture but not necessarily your own—and into your authentic energy needs. When you are living by less authentic influencers, you are doing your Self little good. In fact, you can bring imbalance and even harm into your life, as well as circulate low quality energy to those around you. The danger: this energy pattern can become a norm of influence that then runs under your radar. At higher risk is that, because it is virtually automatic, you start to believe that this (the new norm) is just the way it is, has to be, and will be for you.

Make listening to your Self a daily priority. At times, this will take more patience than others. You may have to dig deeper and listen more carefully in order to find what's triggering a particular obsession. Nevertheless, I encourage you to do so.

Tell yourself that you are exploring the possibility of sparkling, new energies that can make a positive and significant difference in your daily life. Tell yourself that they will lead to greater satisfaction and meaning in your life.

Then tell yourself to reflect. Sometimes reflection and rumination seem alike. The difference is that reflection will steer you toward solution, but rumination will keep you stuck in the problem. So ask yourself: *Am I working the problem or the solution?* Look at the micro picture, then the macro. Now ask: *What's holding me back, and how might I challenge that and get flowing again?*

I knew someone who was extremely reluctant to confront a coworker's off-color and hurtful joking around. His hesitancy stemmed from growing up in a family where there was a lot of emotive criticism—often in the form of vulgar language. He didn't like this crass talk, but he didn't do anything to voice his objections, and his family's aggressive language continued. Similarly, he was trapped into putting up with his coworders' hurtful jokes until he was ready to introspect and dig to expose the energy patterns that were holding him back. In the end, by using the energy of Universal Virtue and making listening to himself a priority, he was able see the energy patterns that had trapped him, see that they were not an accurate representation of who he was—his true Self—use his reasoning to let them go, and respond in a way that brought his work situation to a peaceful and successful resolution.

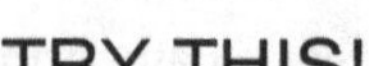

TRY THIS!

When you feel yourself caught in a chain of obsessions, step back and take a close look at what's going on with you. Identify where the gridlock is rooted, and consider what you can do to clear the root problem. If an answer isn't immediately available, you may want to try talking things out with a friend or a professional. Alternately, it may be that you simply need to do more introspection or gather more information from a wider range of sources. Consider how long you have been thinking and feeling like this. Is there any evidence in your life's history that would support such thoughts and feelings? Are these thoughts and feelings functional? Are they reasonable? Are they reliable?

As you dig deeper, consider what really matters to you and to others. Ask yourself: *Do I need to be more honest and forward with myself or others? Do I need to be more creative?*

Now, visualize again how you might clear your gridlock. Think about what mental activity needs to be suppressed and what needs activation. Take action.

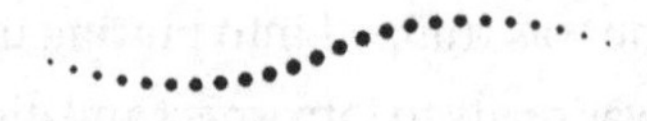

Use Music and Natural Sound

As we've discussed before, your brain loves music and rhythm, and you can learn to use both to reboot your energy and change your mood. Music can also calm and then energize you when obsession or rumination discombobulates you. Simply choose a calming song to help slow down your mind, and help you focus and shut out outside distractions. Then use an upbeat song to inject some energy and restart your mind.

You will also find that different music and sound combinations work in different situations, so experiment with finding songs that sooth or direct your energy in a particular way. Or if you don't want to be directed by anything, try using white noise. It can suppress negativity and help you feel into your place of balance. Natural sounds can work this way too if you know of ones that will have a balancing effect on you, shutting off distractors and activating your focus in a direction of calm and alert.

Use Art

Art works in a similar way to music, controlling obsessions and rebooting your mind to think more positively.

It is always good to have your own self-prescription prepared in advance. But if you are just starting, you can make the discovery process itself part of your reward—especially if you begin with the expectation of finding a new way to re-energize your mind. Consider going to museums and galleries to discover what types of art you respond to most positively, or look at images online or in an art book. You may like to make an album of your favorites and place it in your home, office, or on your cellphone—so you can carry your self-prescription with you everywhere.

TRY THIS!

The next time you find yourself obsessing, treat yourself to a great novel you've been wanting to read that will send you the positive messages and motivation(s) you need to take your mind away from obsessing and toward a solution more quickly. The more you have wanted to read it, the better. Or watch a great movie you have wanted to see but haven't had time for. Before reading the novel or watching the movie, use your power of expectation to anticipate those parts you think will be spectacular. This will amplify their effect with a rewarding cascade of feel-good hormones when you get to those particular scenes. Try feeling into the energy of a character that embodies the energy you think you may need. By recognizing and feeling it, you can use this energy to bring you to a place of peace and balance.

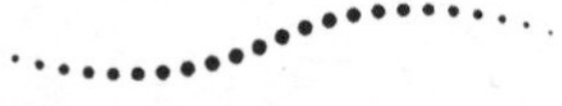

Tai Chi and Yoga

Use energy movement in combination with music and meditation (or solely) to achieve balance from an obsessing or ruminating mind. Tai chi and yoga, unlike other forms of movement, work especially well. Both of these disciplines are, in part, meant to help you flow deeper into the quietness of your mind, and detach from the low quality energies that drive you into circular thinking and feeling. Like the athlete who must suppress elements of her mind that will dull her performance while bringing to the fore those that will put her on the fast track to optimum performance, feel into the energy of your movements, and allow your mind restore to its natural, original state.

Empty Mind

There will be instances when, like the athlete about to compete or the politician about to address an audience, you will find that you do not have the time necessary to stop your mind from obsessing. When this is the case, the only way through is to totally stop thinking—empty your mind of all negative feelings and put all your energy toward being mindful.

The Buddha said, "Truth comes in between breaths." When I was a young martial artist, I thought that this literally meant breath—as in breathing. So I, unfortunately, got tagged repeatedly on the mats. I had a lot to learn.

Most beginning martial artists are obsessed with scoring points or tagging their opponents when sparring; I was no different in that regard. The more time I spent thinking about it, however, the more I seemed to get tagged. I soon figured out that I was losing because I was thinking too much and obsessing about the points being scored. I was pretty thoughtful but not very mindful.

Martial arts are a great teacher of mindfulness because you have to learn not to think obsessively or you will get tagged, almost immediately. In fact, the more you think, the more vulnerable you become—not to mention the more you can be effectively manipulated once your partner knows what you are obsessing over. It's one of the oldest tricks in the book: if a martial artist knows that all you want to do is strike at him, he can just open an irresistible target to you. But now that he knows exactly where you are going to be striking, he can easily block and counter you. This is how the advanced practitioner manipulates the novice. And of course, the trick is used in many other disciplines—politics, advertising, and so on—not just martial arts.

Controlling obsessions in sport isn't easy, but one day, most martial arts students step back and manage to resist their urge to think-think-think. Instead, they relax, shake off all dysfunctional urges and thoughts, and just pay attention. Then, right in front of them—big as a billboard—comes a real target. They execute a move—the right and best one—and nail their target easily, letting their procedural skill kick in the way it is supposed to—automatically, effortlessly. This is a great eye-opener for most martial artists, so they, of course, want to repeat it. And little by little as they begin to trust in the process, it gets easier to knock off obsessive thoughts and feelings, and just stay in the flow.

Martial arts practices sparring situations for the distinct purpose of quickening this procedure and making it more effortless. The good news is that you can incorporate empty mind in all daily tasks, whether you practice martial arts or not.

What Buddha meant by "in between breaths" was in between thoughts. Your true targets in life come in between thoughts—in between what you think is going to happen (or you can make happen). Your formula remains the same: step back, quit thinking, get mindful, wait until your window of opportunity opens, do what is best, rinse, and repeat. This pattern will help you stay in a flowing state of mind more naturally and automatically.

Mind-Body Works

Changes in the mind will change the brain, and changes in the body will change the mind. So if, for instance, every time you begin to ruminate about your job, you practice a strategic distraction or work out instead, you can reprogram your body in that situation and make changes in your mind as a result.

Remember, your body is a vessel and can only hold so much energy. By focusing your body on some task instead of allowing your mind to ruminate, you are removing your dysfunctional energy and replacing it with good. The simpler this task is, the better. Sweeping a floor, doing dishes, or watering flowers will do the trick. I love these simple chores for the easy organized energy they help contain. Afterward, use your renewed energy to power something else you truly need to be doing in your life, such as tending to finances, reading, or doing the shopping. Let these real needs distract you from ruminations in a positive way. Once you get a bit of that done (which will feel good in and of itself), reward yourself.

Exercises and Practices

1. The next time you feel caught in a cycle of repetitive thought, acknowledge that your mind is caught in an energy trap of circular thinking. Name it and feel it. Then relax your mind and body. You know the feeling of cessation—acknowledge that difference. Empty your mind, and tell yourself you are headed toward that feeling.

2. Acknowledge that your urge to obsess is a trap. Give yourself permission to delay any more obsessive thoughts or actions. Instead, get involved in another activity just long enough to help you energetically shift into a place of more balance. At moments like these, an individual I know likes to turn on the radio to find an appealing piece of music and dance rigorously or play air guitar or keyboards.

3. When you find yourself stuck in an energy trap, acknowledge that, then find a quiet place and relax. Visualize a scene from your past when you were doing something athletic. See everything as though you are looking through an orange lens. If you don't like the feeling of orange, make it white or green or whatever you wish. Breathe in slowly, taking the entire picture inward through your lens. Circulate this positive energy in color through all three levels of your consciousness. Feel into it. Now start a second orbit of energy, looping it downward from your highest spiritual mind and back. With a little practice, you can circulate both simultaneously.

10

USING ENERGY TO ENHANCE PHYSICAL STRENGTH

Without passion, you don't have energy;
without energy, you have nothing!

—Donald Trump

When you think of enhancing strength, your mind may go to the athletic endeavors you enjoy, such as rock climbing, golf, or yoga. Or you may think about various things you do throughout your day that require different levels of strength. For many people, this is also a list of tasks including anything from working outdoors to working at a desk or computer.

Strength means different things to us at different phases in our lives. I remember (with a smile) when our children were newborns and I had to develop a new strength that facilitated going through many tasks while holding a child in one arm. I also remember having to stop playing my violin regularly back then because of all the new demands on my time. When I was ready to get back into it, however, I realized just how much strength is involved in playing such a small instrument. And it took a while to rebuild that strength.

Aging will bring different demands on your strength as well. I know several individuals who are enjoying a beautiful longevity in which strength means being able to live in their own home and maneuver about the premises and elsewhere on their own. Some of these people have told me that their goal is to maintain just enough strength in their arms to be able to do those basic tasks that enable them to feed and care for themselves.

Some people, regardless of age, are focusing on gaining and maintaining the strength necessary to recuperate from illness or surgeries and get back in the saddle.

Other times the desire for more strength is more specifically targeted. People look for more strength in their legs, core, arms, or wrists. Many musicians train for hand and finger strength. A martial artist may strengthen her "funny bone" to the point that she can split a cinder block with a single strike, or strengthen her forearms so that she can painlessly strike solid oak—or even iron—at almost full bore.

Obviously, there are many ways in which we may define and interpret the need for enhanced strength in our lives. However, although I acknowledge that strength training can be achieved through all athletics (including weight training) and I advocate for these, I consider them, within the scope of this book, as complementary to cultivating and tapping into various natural energies that enhance your strength for specific life tasks or goals. There are, however, certain activities that overlap with what we consider athletics, (such as yoga and tai chi) that are designed philosophically and scientifically for the purpose of cultivating energy flow within and through your entire being of body-mind-spirit.

Our approach in this chapter will offer a variety of tools you can use to customize a strength-enhancing program to suit your daily and long-range needs. In doing this, we will focus on how a person's greatest strength—again, as we are defining it here—will come from the synchronization, concentration, and execution of a person's internal and external energy sources.

Believe You Can Do It

Powering up for any task involves believing you can do it. You have to believe you have what it takes to get the job done. If this means the strength and know-how, then you have to believe you've got it or can accrue it. Like the karate practitioner visualizing his fist having already broken through a board before striking it, your strength will be fired by your belief that you can accomplish your task.

One thing you can do to build up your confidence is to visualize having completed your task. Think of a previous time when you've pumped up the motivation and power to complete the same or a similar task; remember how you felt during and afterward. Reflecting in this way connects you with a successful energy template you've already generated and can use to succeed again. As you visualize this template, be sure to tell yourself you can indeed do it again. Doing all of this will generate the right mind-set and give you the strength to complete the task at hand.

However, just as this confident mind-set enables you to succeed, the opposite mind-set can block your energy and deplete your strength.

Perhaps one of the greatest examples of this kind of self-defeating mind-set was the historic world-boxing championship in Kinshasa, Zaire, 1974, known as the "Rumble in the Jungle," between world-champion George Foreman and Muhammad Ali. This was the match in which Ali debuted what became known as his "rope-a-dope" technique. Foreman, younger than Ali and thought to be the stronger, enjoyed his reputation as one of the best knockout punchers ever in boxing. Yet he was psychologically deflated by Ali's rope-a-dope tactic. Ali's strategy was to take Foreman's punches while leaning against the ropes and taunting him—as if his strikes had no power. By the eighth round, Foreman was drained of energy and mentally weary. With only a few seconds left in the round, Foreman took a hit and fell onto the canvas for a count of nine. Although Foreman did manage to get up, the referee called the bout, giving Ali the win and the championship with a technical knockout.

Know What You're Getting Into

Knowledge of a task goes a long way. Several years ago, I had the pleasure of working in the dojo with a petite young woman who weighed ninety pounds and had serious vision loss for which she needed the assistance of a guide dog throughout the day. None of this had stopped her from earning a black belt in Chinese kenpo as well as a black belt in jiujitsu. One afternoon, as her seeing-eye dog lay in one of the corners of our room, she was sparring with a black-belt male of over six feet. After only a few moments, he had managed to block one of her kicks and had lifted her off the ground, so that she was over his head. He was showing off because everyone knew she was highly skilled and had already beaten most of the men. But he wasn't going to have that. So he continued to lift her when, all of the sudden, she wrapped her legs in what we call a *figure four* around his neck and cranked the extended leg, like a wrench, dropping him to the mat in seconds.

He was bigger and stronger, but her amount of muscle worked just fine to defeat him in an instant. Why? Because as soon as he placed his hands on her, he abandoned the kicking and boxing world and entered the grappling world, where she had superior knowledge and skill. Over the years, she had used informed power to create automatic procedures that she could launch in a flash to achieve her desired outcome.

What I am saying is that knowing what you are trying to do will not necessarily give you all the strength you need, but it will help you issue the strength you have quickly, correctly, and with more power. And this can make all the difference.

This knowledge doesn't just apply to sports. If, for example, you don't have the strength to sit in a chair and type for as long as you need to, learning about the mechanics of the act and muscle groups involved may help. You may choose to strengthen your wrists and forearms, and make yourself mindful of how you are positioning your feet and holding your shoulders, neck, and chest. You may also discover that a five- to ten-minute mediation, practiced twice throughout the day, helps loosen you up, giving you the additional strength and endurance to accomplish your goal.

I highly recommend following a good energy trail when you discover one. For example, if you find that better posture helps your typing strength and endurance, make tai chi or yoga movement part of your daily routine in the morning, evening, or both. These will affect your performance throughout the day.

Condensing Energy

An important technique in mind-body medicine is *condensing energy*, which enables you to summon energy from all your resources and compress it into explosive strength. We believe that where the mind goes, your energy will follow. This helps you route your full being energy to where it will do you the most good. Martial arts and traditional Asian movement use condensed energy, relying on what is termed *fa jin* (explosive power) in a variety of their techniques. One of the most famous of these techniques was popularized by Bruce Lee with his famous one-inch punch, showing how you could summon great physical power and issue it effectively into a target an inch or less away.

A martial arts master once demonstrated this famous one-inch punch on me. Before he did, he gathered a handful of thick phone books and handed three of them to me. They were to protect me, he said.

He instructed me to hold the phone books flat against my abdomen, like a shield.

"You won't get hurt," he assured me. "The phone books will absorb the shock."

Then, from no more than an inch away, he executed a punch that, after contact, he retracted instantly. For a second, I felt only the thrust of the shot, but then I felt a curious swell of energy about the size of a golf ball traveling through my abdomen. It felt uncanny. It felt as though the amassed energy could explode into pain at any moment. But it never did. It was as though the energy had been injected into me and passed straight through, without leaving a mark. Later, he explained that the energy I felt was his energy passing through; if I hadn't had the phone books to absorb some of it, I could have been seriously injured. This is the kind of strike that can pass through the area of initial contact yet leave a bruise on someone's back.

Bruce Lee, though athletically built, had a relatively small frame and was a few inches below the average in height. Nonetheless, his one-inch punch showed that there was more to strength and issuing power than size and muscle. So what else is there that allows Lee and other martial artists that kind of strength in the face of others who are a lot bigger in size?

In terms of kung fu and karate (and athletics in general), the activation, precision, and coordination of body movement plays a significant role. Bruce Lee powered up his punch, for instance, through precise coordination of all his movements, from his feet to his head—twists, turns, extensions, and a final flick of the wrist before impact—as well as their speed and timing. In other words, he executed the technique with optimum precision.

In 2012, in the Oxford University Journal, *Cerebral Cortex*, Dr. R. E. Roberts wrote of a study he had conducted looking into just why martial arts masters like Lee were able to generate such power.[1] One of the things Roberts found was that practicing martial arts increases the brain's *white matter*, which forms the connective (communicative) tissue between various regions of the brain. This change in brain matter is able to speed up communication among the brain areas that involve coordination and power of movement. For this reason, many martial arts practitioners (as well as yoga, tai chi, chi kung practitioners, and the like) predictably report feeling a new sense of strength and more coordination in almost everything they do daily—from the most mundane tasks to the most athletic, and everything in between. Not only that but they have more endurance for all these activities, and they experience a more flowing mind-set. This matches my own experience (in chapter 1) of stacking wood with more robust and flowing energy early in my martial arts experiences.

Therefore, the martial arts practitioner creates a win-win situation by improving neuroconnectivity via physical training and improving physical training via quicker communication within the brain. But do you have to be a martial artist to activate explosive and coordinated energy processes in your own mind and body? The answer is not at all. Yet we can learn from the martial arts and from research such as that conducted by Dr. Roberts.

Looking at what we've said so far, which is solely in physiological realm, there are three factors you need to consider when condensing energy to build strength.

First, you need to relax. The softer you are, the less tension you hold in your muscles (and mind), and the faster and smoother you can move.

Then put your whole body into the action. If you are typing, for example, consider the movement (or stillness, flexibility, calmness) of other areas of your body that will optimize your goal. Find your optimum posture for your specific activity and practice it. Like the martial artist, you can commit the full posture and movement to memory, and use that memory until you begin to fall into this optimum pattern quickly and automatically.

Lastly, learn to empty your mind and relax after you have issued power. This is important because, as with the martial artist's issuance of an explosive punch, you need to ward off recoil, which can drain your energy and even hurt you. So if you are lifting a heavy weight, after you have done your rep, take a moment to breathe and rest before you exert again.

Life is full of situations that call for intense, informed power. By following these steps, you can synchronize your energies and learn to deal with these situations smoothly and effectively—and avoid potential backlash.

Using Visualization to Condense Energy into Strength

A tai chi master I know used to work two weeks in a hospital each summer, helping patients who required rehab after various surgeries. His mission was to use the high-quality, nourishing energy of tai chi to put them in a more positive mind-set, but also to help them recuperate more quickly and regain their strength. Most of the patients had very weak body strength and movement. When I asked him how he taught them tai chi, considering their condition—as some were bedridden or bound to chairs—he said it was all done in the mind, through visualization. In essence, these patients practiced the same movement you or I would practice outdoors or on the mats in a studio, only they went through the postures and movements in their mind. Nonetheless, he maintained that the results were consistently good: patients generally became more positive and energetic, and increased their physical strength.

Activities like this often work because visualization activates the same parts of the brain that a specific movement does. For example, imagining that you are moving the fingers on your right hand activates the same brain area that physically moving them does. You can use visualizations that enable you to focus on various areas of the body you wish to strengthen, working them out (electrochemically), or making them stronger or healing them. But you can additionally learn to use visualization to compress the energy within and around you into a powerful "bundle" and route it to where you need, such as to your foot or to your neck.

Although holistic medicines have scientifically practiced and honed techniques for using the mind to considerably strengthen and even heal the body for millennia, there has been interesting evidence put forth by various conventionally trained scientists in the past few years that substantiates this practice from their perspective. We are delighted to see this and hope to see more of it in the future, as such research helps us all to better understand the workings of the mind-body connection and how we can regulate it.

In a 2013 article titled "Mental Imagery May Hasten Recovery after Surgery" at ScientificAmerican.com, two such studies are cited. The first, which first appeared in the December 2012 issue of the *Scandinavian Journal of Medicine and Science in Sports*, showed how a group of individuals "that practiced guided imagery [visualizations of the healing process] exhibited greater improvements in knee stability [after Anterior Cruciate Ligament (ACL) Surgery] and reduced levels of stress hormones."[2] ACL surgery involves reconstruction or repair of the ligament. (Such ACL tears are rampant in athletes.)

The other experiment was conducted on patients scheduled for gallbladder removal. First appearing in the February 2012 issue of *Brain, Behavior, and Immunity*, this experiment showed that "compared with [the] control group, participants who practiced imagery [visualization] reported a larger reduction in stress, and their wounds showed signs of greater collagen deposition and faster healing."[3]

In another study titled, "From Mental Power to Muscle Power—Gaining Strength by Using the Mind," conducted at the Lerner Research

Institute departments of Biomedical Engineering and Physical Medicine and Rehabilitation in Cleveland, Dr. V. K. Ranganathan and colleagues showed that you can gain significant muscle strength by mental training alone—results that are quite compelling. "This finding suggests that mental-training-induced neural adaptations have long-lasting effect that is reflected by continuously enhanced strength output."[4] Dr. Ranganathan goes on to say that "mental training perhaps leaves neural traces, similar to those following motor learning, that are [a] long-lasting and almost unforgettable, such as those like riding a bicycle, ice skating, and swimming."[5]

But you need patience. What is also necessary for successful use of visualization is a lot of repetition and daily practice.

TRY THIS!

Visualize moving energy within and throughout your body with your breathing—in-breaths and out-breaths. You may like to imagine this energy as bright white fog or light.

Breathe in and visualize yourself drawing energy from your extremities to your dan tien (center of your body) and condensing it tightly into a smaller and smaller space. Route this condensed energy back through your arms, hands, legs, and feet with your out-breaths. Feel into the flowing energy. Imagine your extremities strengthening.

Now imagine an exercise in which you are using the specific extremities you want to strengthen, such as digging in a garden. Feel into your arms slowly. Feel your condensed energy entering them. You may feel sensations of warmth or heat. Let this soothe your joints and muscles. Visualize it warmer if that is more comfortable—or cooler. Do as many reps as you are comfortable doing.

Remember to stay softly focused and calm, and push your "clear" button after. Experiment with this process, using sound and colors (or even a mental narrative) that enhance your sensations of strength. Create new activities for yourself, focusing on the same areas. Remember: repetition is key.

Power Massage

Several mind-body medical practices involve forms of massage that target specific energy points (acupuncture points) on the body. This practice is to help you open up access to energy channels that contain and issue the energy you need at specific times. It can also strengthen your overall operating energy. Although these methodologies and energy points may be known by different names, depending on who uses them and their own discipline, they are well known throughout the world of holistic medicine and arts. I enjoy them all because they can deliver instant results and only take a few minutes to perform.

The following is a list of my own personal favorites, which I practice and have taught many other individuals to use. You don't have to use the entire regimen for your own cultivation and practice; use those that feel best for you. That may include just one or a few daily, or the entire list as needed. Do what's comfortable.

The Bubbling Well is an energy point located at the bottom of each foot that is capable of releasing streams of strengthening energy almost instantly throughout the body. To access it, begin in either a seated or standing position. Turn your left foot so that it is bottom up. Then, holding it in place with your left hand, massage the center of your foot with the thumb of your right hand. If it is more comfortable for you to use your right hand to massage, do that. Then massage the same area of your right foot. You should feel this energy streaming through your body. Take a slow breath and exhale.

There are energy points that run in a line down your forearms that often get blocked. Unlocked, the line supplies clean, strong energy to your arms and other parts of your body. I recommend opening this energy line daily, as it can power you up for anything—from athletics to household chores—and can make you feel stronger in general. To open this line, slow down and deepen your breathing. Using the tips of the fingers on your right hand, start tapping about two inches above your elbow, and tap down the top of your forearm and back up. Do this a few times (you will "feel" the precise line as you do). Then follow the same procedure for your other arm. Take a slow breath and exhale.

This same procedure can also be used on your legs to power up your energy: Slow down and deepen your breathing. Follow the same procedure as above, except tap along the energy points lined down the outer side of each leg—from just below your hip to your ankle, and back up. With very little practice, you will find the precise line. Take a slow breath and exhale. You may prefer to make a fist and use your knuckle joints instead of fingertips for this one. Try both and pick what's best for you.

Another energy point is located in the center of your chest. When unblocked, this point sends strong calming and revitalizing energy to your heart and throughout the rest of you. To unblock this point, make a gentle fist with your right hand and gently tap with the palm side of your fist on your breastbone several times (or use your fingertips, whichever feels gentler). Slow down and deepen your breathing. Feel your energy and strength powering up, but don't overdo it. Take a slow breath and exhale.

Just underneath your collarbone, you will find two energy points, one on either side. Unblocked, these stream energy to your lungs and throat; and affect the quality of your breathing, increase calmness, and invigorate you. Take in a deep and slow breath. Exhale slowly. Position your index and middle fingers of your left and right hands, respectively, on the energy point located about an inch underneath and to the side (toward your shoulders) the left and right tips of your collarbone. Tap (or rub) gently with your fingertips below each end of your collarbones. Take a slow breath and exhale.

There are two energy points located behind your neck—on either side—just below the base of your skull. Unblocked, these stream energy to your mind and brighten your consciousness. To open them, intertwine the fingers of your left and right hands. Take a deep and slow breath. Exhale slowly. Hold and place your palms (with fingers still intertwined) against the back of your head, then straighten your back and head. Gently push your head back into your palms. Gently tap your neck three times (only three) with your thumbs—again, just below the base of your skull. Take a slow breath and exhale.

Once you are enjoying the increased energy and quality effects of opening some or all of these energy points, try condensing the energy you accrue from them (individually or collectively), routing it within your mind-body to where it will do you the most good.

Muscle Up with Your Playlist

As we've discussed, music with different rhythms and tempos can do wonders for your mood and energy. Similarly, it can boost your endurance, and make work and workouts seem easier. Experiment with songs with different BPMs and rhythms to see which give you the best energy boost. As you do so, pick songs with lyrics that send you the message you need to be hearing on a particular day. Remember that not every song works for every situation. A song that gives you the energy you need to complete a hard workout may not be the best song to listen to when you need to get energized before giving a speech.

Energy Drills

Energy drills incorporate rhythmic *psychomotor movement* intended to help empty your mind; fill you with great, positive, and enduring energy; and strengthen your body. Because they tap into the mind's love of patterns, these rhythms ingrain in your memory and are easy to bottle up, so to speak, for when you need them later. The following drills—one solo, the other with a partner—can be practiced either in the morning or the evening. Only use these once a day, and add reps as you feel comfortable—but don't overdo either drill. Too much will strain your joints and ligaments.

The first solo drill is known as the *hubud.* This is an energy drill used in Filipino as well as other martial arts. Stand about a foot away from a smooth wall and face it. Relax yourself completely, especially your shoulders. Place your right foot forward. Bend your knees slightly and relax your hips. Gently bend your right elbow and place your right forearm against the wall, so that it is directly in front of you and perpendicular to the ground. Don't push against the wall; just let your arm rest there. Make a fist with your right hand; then, with your left hand (open palm), reach across to the thumb of your right hand and, very lightly, without touching the wall with any part of your right (or left) hand or forearm (leave only your elbow touching), pull the right forearm down to the nine o'clock position. Let go of your right hand and rotate your right forearm, still keeping your elbow to the wall, back to the twelve o'clock position, very gently tapping the wall with the back of your fist. This should all be done softly and fluidly. Repeat a few times.

After you get the hang of the movements as described in the paragraph above; do them nonstop a few times, using the same hand-arm motions as you did, only without actually touching hands or tapping the wall. Just your elbow should be touching the wall, nothing else.

Keep this rotation movement going, and count each time your fist comes back to the twelve o'clock position—1, 2, 3, 4, then 1, 2, 3, 4, and so on. Feel into the energy of movement but also into the rhythm itself. Count out loud, when appropriate. (Hearing the rhythm aloud will better ingrain it in your mind.) Whenever you want to access that energy throughout the day, all you have to do is visualize yourself doing the hubud and count the rhythm in your mind. As you get comfortable with the routine, you can do more reps and pick up speed. But don't get sloppy with the pattern, and don't overdo it. For even more energy, use a 1-2, 1-2 count.

When you finish, regulate your breathing and condense the energy you have gained. Circulate this luxurious force throughout your entire body-mind-spirit. Take a few slow and deep breaths, and feel this force strengthening you.

The second drill, which is done with a partner, is known as the *Smashing Four Star.* Stand facing your partner, about two feet apart. Cross your right forearms so the top side of your forearm is touching that of your partner midway between the wrist and the elbow, forming an "X" at about six o'clock between you. Gently tap your forearms together, then separate and raise them in a clockwise motion, bringing your right arms to twelve o'clock, and tap forearms again. Draw your right arms back to your sides, and do the same "X" with your left arms. Repeat this action, alternating right and left arms, for one to two minutes. As you get comfortable, you can pick up speed and extend the time. The additional speed will give you additional energy, but never overdo it. And remember to tap lightly—don't hurt anyone.

When you finish, regulate your breathing and condense the energy you have gained. Then circulate this luxurious force throughout your entire body-mind-spirit. Take a few slow and deep breaths, and feel this force strengthening you.

Cultivate and Store Your Energy

There are three easy ways you can cultivate and store energy throughout the day, and I highly recommend that you add all three to your daily routine. You can start with one at a time, but attaining the full regimen should be your goal.

The first and easiest way (for many people) to cultivate energy and increase strength is to start off your day with the physical exercise of your choice. As we discussed earlier, your body will begin to automatically boost your energy daily and on schedule if you do this. Use exercise activities you like (or think you will like), as they will loop into your mind-body reward system, and give you that extra motivation to commit.

Regular cardiovascular exercise works great for this. Nutritionist Samantha Heller said in an interview with WebMD that "your body rises up to meet the challenge for more energy [resulting from exercise] by becoming stronger . . . It all begins with tiny organs called mitochondria. Located in our cells, they work like tiny power plants to produce energy."[6] Heller explains that some of your energy does come from diet, and not eating enough can power down your metabolism. Yet "the number of mitochondria you have—and thus your ability to produce energy—is affected by your daily activity."[7]

The beauty of this is that it means you can create an automatic strengthening loop of energy for yourself. Opening each day with physical activity you enjoy will not only strengthen you but fine-tune your body's capacity to power up automatically, upon need. Try to exercise for twenty minutes to an hour daily. If you miss a day, don't worry about doubling up; just be consistent over time. Immediately after physical exercise, condense and circulate the energy you have collected. As you feel your surges of strength, feel into the energy. Familiarize yourself with what it feels like to be in this condition. This way you can use your mind to re-create it for you later.

Mindfulness is the second component you want to add to your daily strengthening practice. You can use this as a strengthening tool right in the middle of activity—exercise and otherwise. Make yourself mindful of where—within you—you need more strength. Then focus on your lower dan tien and, using your breath, pull in the energy from your extremities, condense it, and route it back where you need it most. If your extremities are consuming energy, use your in-breaths to draw from your environment. Consider your immediate surroundings and all three levels of body (physical), mind, and spirit. Condense and circulate the energy. The more you practice this strengthening energy loop, the faster and more automatic the process will become. Eventually, your mind-body will kick in all on its own.

On certain occasions, or if you cannot engage in physical activity, you may substitute the following technique for exercise: Guide the entire activity in your mind and body with images, and condense and circulate the energy it cultivates. The more you have combined this activity with real-time exercise in the past, the more effective it will be. I'd like to gently suggest starting today, so that you can have your strengthening energy in storage for when you need it.

Energy meditation is also something you want to add to your list of daily to-dos. Any energy-heightening meditations we have discussed so far—and throughout the rest of this book—will work. My personal favorite is transferring fresh, clean, vibrant energy downward, through all three levels of consciousness, using meditation in combination with music, sound, scent, and visualization for an even greater effect.

Remember, there is only so much energy you can hold. And negative energy is disempowering. Constant drain and consumption will leave you weak and fatigued. So vanish the negative, plug the drain, and replenish with high quality energy that will strengthen you.

Again, feeling into all of these energies and getting to know what your body feels like under their influence is important. This is what enables you to put them aside so that you can draw on them later, condense them, and issue them as power.

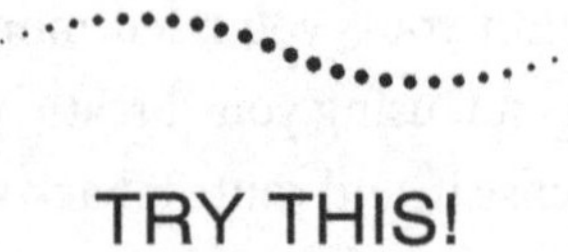

TRY THIS!

Relax and concentrate on your lower dan tien. Keep your hands there so you can better direct your breath to it. Breathe deeply and smoothly while counting to ten; hold your breath to the same brisk count; and then release it, also to the same count. Listen to the sound of your breath. Let that sound ingrain like musical sounds and rhythms in your mind.

Now draw your breath down to your lower dan tien, and feel into the energy gathering there. Draw up energy from the earth. Feel into it as it is entering your body through the bottoms of your feet. Let that energy also gather in your lower dan tien. Likewise, draw the energy above you into your body through your *upper dan tien* (located at the crown of your head). Let it flow and gather where you are holding your hands. Use deep breathing to route this energy where you wish it to go in your body. If you need a little help, touch your fingers to areas you are intending to invigorate, and strengthen and target your breath there. Feel into the clean, nutritious energy strengthening you.

When you finish, regulate your breathing and condense the energy you have gained. Then circulate this luxurious force throughout your entire body-mind-spirit. Take a few slow and deep breaths, and feel this force strengthening you. Imagine yourself ten feet tall and ready to take on anything. Feel your power. Feel your strength.

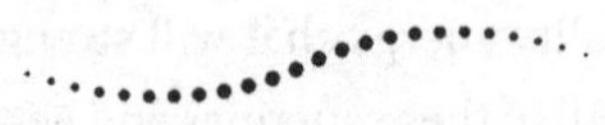

Exercises and Practices

1. Be mindful of the rhythms you experience while exercising, such as while jogging or dancing. Count out your most activating and strengthening rhythmic patterns to yourself—e.g., 1-2-3-4, 1-2-3-4, or 1-2, 1-2. Later, anytime after the exercise, reflect on the activity and count out the rhythms to yourself, feeling into their energy. Visualize yourself performing a specific daily task as you count, and feel into the energy. You can even visualize yourself in a new task you'll tackle sometime in the future. The idea is to attach the rhythm to a specific endeavor and commit it to memory through your visualization. Once you have ingrained the pattern in your memory, you have it available to give you a fast and fresh boost of strength anytime, anywhere—whenever you need it. All you have to do is hear it in your mind. Remember, this practice adds more white matter to your brain, quickening communication and coordination between those brain areas needed for particular motor skills. Prepare now, in advance, and you'll be all set in times of need.

2. Use visualization. Relax and regulate your breathing. Use your in-breaths to condense your energy until you visualize it as being the size of a dime. Use three out-breaths to guide it to where you need it in your body. Feel into it, using breathing to draw energy from all extremities, and your lower and upper dan tien. Do this for no more than three breaths. Then release it with an out-breath. With practice, this energizer will become automatic and work more effectively.

3. Use your brain's language and emotional circuits. Have on hand a few power words that put you in a positive and focused mind-set, and are task appropriate—words like *strong*, *flow*, *explode*, *go-go-go*.

The best ones will be those you like that have an emotional tie to a time when you are on top of your game.

4. Find a recording of a drum solo that makes you feel strong, alert, energized. Add the piece to your cell phone or other electronic playlists so that you can have it as needed. The more you listen to the drumbeat, the more this rhythm ingrains. The more it ingrains, the faster and more effectively it will work to give you the strength you need for the specific situation(s) you attach it to.

5. Increase your brain's motor communication. Relax and regulate your breathing. Put on a piece of music that you find stimulating. Close your eyes and visualize yourself doing a particular exercise. Use as many of your senses as possible. Imagine yourself as performing on top of your game. This activity can be helpful for anyone trying to pump up for a wide range of activities, and for those who may be sedentary.

11

USING ENERGY TO IMPROVE MEMORY

Memory is like a spiderweb that catches new information.
The more it catches, the bigger it grows.
And the bigger it grows, the more it catches.

—Joshua Foer

Memory plays a large role in your ability to create new energy circuits to give you high quality energy for the very specific things you want to do. But it also plays a role in why we lose energy—even unconsciously. It can block your energy resources too. So, improving your memory can be a great facilitator of happiness and good living—a storage tank generating and recycling many life problems.

Your memory is an incredible thing. Often, all it takes is hearing just a few words or notes from a song you last heard years ago to recall the whole piece. Similarly, just the slightest fragrance can send you back to a room in your grandma's house during the holidays, when you were a child.

In contrast, you can walk from one room of your house into another and forget what you went in there for. Who hasn't gone out to the store for a very specific item; bought a cart full of groceries; and then halfway home, realized you forgot the very item you went there to purchase?

Don't worry, lapses of memory happen to all of us. While there are times when we can remember some things with tremendous accuracy and speed, at other times, we forget things we think we know well. We can learn from our moments of clear, fast memory and use this information to help us enter them more freely.

What Memory Is

We sometimes talk about memory as if it were a filing cabinet in our heads—as if, when we recall a piece of information, a drawer pops open and out comes the whole picture or a whole experience. Memory at the physical level, however, operates more like a process, electrochemically fetching information from various areas of the brain and creating a single, unified representation.

Imagine, for the moment, looking up at a star-studded sky with streaks of light connecting clusters of stars. Your brain retrieving a memory would look something like that, as it passes a signal activating an ensemble of *neurons* for data.

This process of retrieving information from your memory explains why, if you are at a concert, you see the "lead guitarist playing a green, electric guitar" rather than a series of separate characteristics, such as: musician, lead guitarist, green, guitar, and playing; you see the experience as one, unified whole. Yet energetically etched in your memory is the name for such an instrument when you encounter it (guitar), a definition for "guitarist" (one who plays a guitar), words for various colors (green), and so on. You are not conscious of the retrieval and integration process you are undergoing because it happens in just milliseconds and *voilà*! There is your perception and image of a "lead guitarist playing a green, electric guitar."

To initiate the process of making a memory, you must first pay attention to the data that comes to you through your senses as opposed to the whole river of information flowing at you second by second.

Sustaining your focus (holding your focus) on certain information sparks the first part of the recording process, which is *encoding* the data into a form your mind and body recognize and put into storage for later use. As previously mentioned, this process is electrochemical, traveling between the spaces (synapses) amid your brain cells and organizing them into a collaboration that, when activated again, will re-create the experience for you. Each time you retrieve the memory, you strengthen this whole chain of activity.

Memory storage lasts from only milliseconds to long-term storage, or what we call long-term memory. You can recall huge amounts of information that is stored in your long-term memory—data from childhood experiences to a painting you saw in a museum, or a piece of jewelry a stranger wore weeks ago that you happened to like a lot. But you can only hold a very limited amount of information in your short-term memory. For example, you catch the title to a great song you hear on the radio on your way home from work. You tell yourself that you will buy the tune for your playlist as soon as you get home. But then you get home and can't recall the title or any detail that would give you a clue to finding the song. Most of us have experienced this kind of memory loss. The information remains in your short-term memory and then naturally vanishes.

How much can this memory bank hold? The magic number seven (as with phone numbers) has been popularized by psychologists and educators as a measurement of how many (or few) items your short-term memory (*working memory*) can retain without stressing out. Its limitations have even been discussed in several comedy routines. One such skit is from comedian Kevin James. He titles the skit "Phone Number Rhythm," poking fun at how little it takes to rock his memory.[1] All it takes to totally interfere with his recalling a phone number is three more digits—the additional three area-code digits—which even get in the way of his ability to write the number down.

You can't focus on every single thing in your environment either, as paying attention to too much can be as detrimental as paying attention to too little. Inhibiting or filtering out certain information and sustaining focus on what you need can help you store information in your long-term memory. By focusing on what is important, you tell your brain that this is the specific material you wish to remember. This process works best when you do it repeatedly. And the more reps you do, the better you will train your brain to more quickly recall the information that you want to remember.

I used this process years ago, when I began learning how to play Irish dance songs on my violin. There were many notes in each of the tunes, but I didn't want to rely on sheet music to play them, so I learned the songs by memorizing a few notes at a time. I started by focusing on a few short lines of melody and practicing them over and over. Then the next day, I focused on adding just a few more; and I kept doing this until I learned a whole song and was able to play it all by memory. Each time I used this learning pattern, I energetically felt rewarded and motivated to learn more says this way.

In the years to come, I would sometimes play the songs only once a year, on St. Patrick's Day, yet I could recall most of the notes immediately. Sometimes, I'd have to go over a section here and there a few times because my recall had slightly deteriorated; but with a few run-throughs, I was up to snuff again—not just with the notes but all the little extras too (like trills and slides, or rocking the bow). Whenever I am trying to commit longer pieces of information to memory, I remind myself of how I learned these songs.

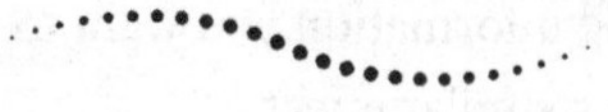

TRY THIS!

Find a power word you can use to strengthen your focus, and repeat it throughout this process. Use your breath to draw energy into your upper and lower dan tiens from your extremities and your external environment. Condense this energy. Circulate it. Repeat this pattern a few times, always chanting your power word. Feel into the incoming and sparkling energy. You will feel alert and calm and balanced.

Use this activity before looking at data you wish to commit to memory, then review the data. Refocus on the information a few times right away, taking a break and repeating the exercise; and approach the information you want to memorize again later on. Repeat this several times. Once you condition this routine, your mind will begin adjusting naturally and faster, using only the power word.

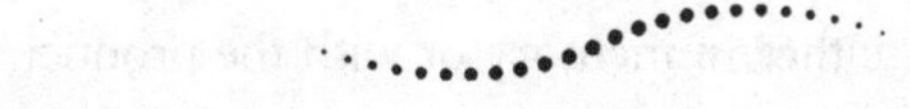

Variety of Detail Gives You Deeper Memory

You can energetically associate information you want to commit to memory with other sensory and even motor detail to give it lasting power. This is because the more intricate your memory, the more storage you activate; and the easier it is for it all to stream into more brain areas.

Executives for television shows, movies, and radio programs have harnessed the energy power of music to trigger deep parts of your memory. These theme songs hold memory so well that you can probably remember several of them from way back in your early youth with ease.

What's more, attaching information you want to remember to any other sensory data can have a similar effect.

Consider scent. You smell freshly mowed grass or the tang of chlorine and you think of summer. Many of us smell pumpkin-patch or apple-orchard scents and we think of autumn; or the scent of certain candles or foods spark holiday memories. But could scent do even more?

A lot of researchers and advertisers think so. This is because, like sound and music, scent has the capacity to bypass your "thinking" brain and shoot straight into your emotional mind-set.

Numbers can sometimes tell part of the story. British newspaper, *The Independent*, for instance, reported that corporate giant, "Nike showed that adding scents to their stores increased intent to purchase by 80 percent; while in another experiment at a petrol station with a mini-mart attached to it, pumping around the smell of coffee saw purchases of the drink increase by 300 percent."[2]

These examples are based on the idea that if you associate scent with the memory of something pleasant and further associate it with a specific product, it will attract you to the merchandise. Of course, if your experience is negative, either in memory or with the product, the marketing ploy won't work.

Visuals work too. Next time you are watching a fast-food ad on television, check out the actors to see if they spark pleasant memories and desires. This method of association is also commonly used with pharmaceutical drug ads, which usually depict people looking pretty good rather than writhing in pain or other malaise—implying this happy, healthy-looking person could be you "on" the pharmaceutical. All you have to do is ask your doctor for a prescription.

Again, attaching information that you want to remember to other information energetically increases memory storage to more than one location, and it strengthens connectivity among synapses. Many times, this process occurs naturally, without your thinking about it. For example, when you visit a place from your past—where you used to work or where you went to school—different rooms trigger various memories of things you did there, in that specific place, long ago. But there is no reason to wait until your mind needs the extra help remembering; start using your associative memory today.

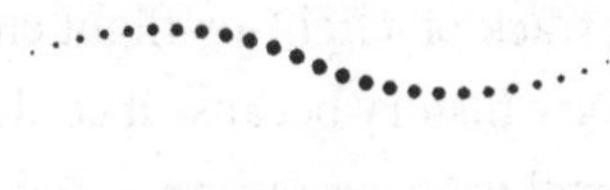

TRY THIS!

Is there a certain scent you have come to associate with working optimally—a scent that makes you feel clear, focused, and happy, with good motivation and memory? If not, create one by joining any specific activity to a specific fragrance. First, identify the activity you wish to energetically enhance by using memory. Then, pick a fragrance and fill your work space with it; use natural substances, such as flowers, or scented candles or oil. Many individuals I know love to review paperwork in a coffee shop. They keep doing this because the "place" has come to work for them consistently. It's not just the caffeine that stimulates them but the scent of roasted coffee that permeates the shop, and perhaps other sensory aspects of the shop itself. You may have such a place that you patronize. Re-creating this fragrance in another space—your home office, for example—can have the same effect. As an alternative, when you are feeling on top of your game for a particular task, attach it to a fragrance you think will be a match. Do this on several occasions. Then use your memory of that fragrance in a targeted environment to boost your performance in the future.

Using Sound

Looking through an evolutionary lens, attaching sound to memory is a very old survival drive that allows you to recognize something by sound, even before you see it. Consider the proverbial tiger-behind-the-bushes example: Your ability to recognize the sound of a hidden tiger, even if only on the fast track of a fight-or-flight emotional response, was important in evolutionary history because it could save your life.

You can use this evolutionary response and attach information to sound to improve memory storage and recall speed. One way is to say the necessary information aloud to yourself a few times, to help you remember. Many ancient traditions and current world traditions use chants and communal repetition of prayers to help individuals drive various scriptural detail into their memory—and ultimately, into their thinking and actions.

For instance, you might use this process when you are in your car, heading to the store to purchase a few items, and have no way of writing a grocery list. Simply saying the items aloud a few times will increase your chances of remembering. Psychologists refer to this as a *phonological loop*. If you are not in a private space, you can use your inner voice to repeat the information in your mind. As with all repetition, this sends your mind the message you want to hold onto the information a while longer.

Recordings of natural sound work as well. A physician I know uses the sound of a campfire to help her reflect before she engages in activities in which memorization will play a role, such as organizing information for a professional interview she will be giving. As she listens to the sound of the campfire, she sends her mind back to when she lived in Italy with her parents as a young girl. She visualizes a sort of mind movie, including people she knew there and specific things she did with them—particularly those with an emotional context, as when she got her first puppy on her seventh birthday. She tries to re-experience as much of the event as possible in all of its assorted detail, including sights, sounds, actions, scents, and emotions—this puts her mind in remembering mode. She practices this for ten to twelve minutes. Afterward, she plays a three minute soundtrack of a waterfall with snapping rapids. This rhythm and tempo works to stimulate her. She augments it with a visualization of a white-water rafting competition she participated in annually with her best friend in college. Feeling refreshed, alert, and calm, with her mind balanced in remembering mode, she turns off the sounds and begins to commit to memory the details for her upcoming interview. She repeats her review of materials a few times. She then goes through the whole regimen (sounds, visualization, and reviewing materials) a few more times during the days leading up to her interview. Her routine helps make long-term memorization possible and successful.

Using Music

It's no wonder that music can play a role in our ability to tap and formulate memories. From our earliest articulations and movements, we learn to sing and dance before we can talk or walk. In terms of memory, we know that infants recognize their mother's voices upon birth. They recognize their mother's approaching footsteps, and can even recognize a song she may have sung or played for them while they were still in the womb. This is a primitive memory skill that bypasses thinking and attaches pleasure to the energy of specific musical sounds.

The ways in which you can use music to improve memory are numerous. One of my daughters loves memorizing important parts of her schoolwork by putting the vital info to the melody of songs she already knows, or even to her own melodies. I know plenty of adults, in fact, who successfully use this technique.

Professional dancers, ice skaters, actors, public speakers, choreographers, and many others use music and sound as a way of memorizing routines—lines, expressions, scenes, as well as spatial and other cues.

Combining sound and rhythm, another individual I know is able to attach information to rap songs she writes for pieces of information she is trying to commit to memory. "The Elements" song by Tom Lehrer is an entertaining example of putting information you want to memorize into a melody.

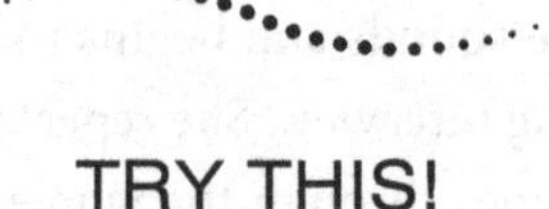

TRY THIS!

This five-minute fix can give you fast recall power during a busy day. Try it right now by finding a place to relax, then pick one of your favorite songs from as far back as you want to remember—childhood, high school. Be sure to pick a song you associate with an emotionally meaningful and soothing time and place.

Visualize a narrative in your mind (a mind movie) that corresponds to the time, place, and music you are listening to. Fill in a great experience you had, using characters and action. Appeal to as many of your senses as you can. Remember, the richer the detail, the more effective your encoding and recall will be. This is a good time to open up a tiny bottle of comforting fragrance that would correspond to the time and place you are remembering. Practice and enjoy this regimen often, to ingrain it in your mind.

The next time you want a general memory boost or you need to memorize something specific, play and feel into the energy of the full-sensory movie in your mind, then approach the material you need to memorize. This will help keep you be calm and focused, and heighten your ability to recall information.

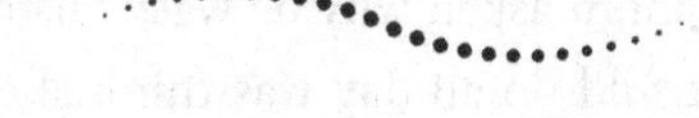

Reasons Why You Lose Memory

We experience memory loss for many reasons, and its symptoms can sometimes overlap. Memory loss may be due to anything from overall physical health, functionality, and development to psychological and spiritual health, functionality, and development. Furthermore, the reason for memory difficulties may lie outside of your body, and they can be difficult to identify.

For example, Benjamin is an elementary school student, and his teacher recently became concerned about his ability to stay focused on classwork. A large part of her concern was centered on how his inattentiveness had affected his ability to draw from memory the information he needed to work on new assignments. She mentioned her concerns to his parents several times.

After weeks of this, Ben's teacher met with his mom and dad to say that he seemed to be digressing academically. She told them Ben couldn't remember important material that she had gone over adequately in class. She was concerned because the material was foundational, and his inability to recall it was now snowballing into a lack of understanding and inability to work on his lessons. She feared, if the pattern continued, he would fall behind and potentially stay behind.

Ben's parents were puzzled, as he seemed quite attentive and able to remember things at home. To test the teacher's observations, Mom read him a story and asked him questions about it. He seemed to like the challenge and maintained interest. And Ben had not had trouble memorizing schoolwork in previous years. What was going on differently this year?

Finally, after extensive questioning, Ben admitted that he was having a hard time remembering things in class because he wasn't listening to his teacher. When his mom asked why he wasn't listening, he explained it was because all he could do all day was think about ways to avoid a couple of boys who were routinely bullying him on the bus after school. Once the school principal took care of the bullying problems, the quality of Ben's performance improved.

As with so many aspects of the body-mind-spirit energy connection, a little knowledge can go a long way in our appreciation, understanding, and success in dealing with a problem.

I go deeper into the complications of memory loss in my book *Can I Have Your Attention?* and discuss a wide range of problems, including Alzheimer's Disease, ADHD, PTSD, endocrine disorders, and so on.[3] But I wish to take a different route for the purpose our discussion here by addressing the annoying, everyday forgetfulness we all experience now and then as we go through our daily routines. Typical, everyday forgetfulness can have many causes, but fortunately, there are energy fixes that you can use to get back on track.

One common cause of everyday forgetfulness is an energy problem. Either you do not have enough overall psychic energy (alertness) or your energy is imbalanced. Here, the principle of yin-yang plays in. For example, you may have too much excitability (yang) or your calm energy (yin) may be too high. When you feel an energy imbalance like this, ask yourself which energy you need to increase or decrease. Then ask yourself if you are being too analytical or placing too much emphasis on productivity and outcome (too much yang), or not enough (yang deficient). You might find that you are being too introspective or putting too much emphasis on creativity (too much yin) or not enough of these (yin deficient). Once you determine the imbalance, use your energy tools to adjust toward a more balanced and optimal mind-set, with improved recall.

Another common cause of forgetfulness is weak focus. You may not be focusing (or focusing long enough) on the information you deem important and want to commit to memory. Remember, focus initiates the storage process. When you feel like your focus is weak, relax and step back. Use one of your power words to refresh and channel your energy. Consider what's important to pay attention to regarding the details of your task. Also, be sure to consider what others see as important. Connect this information to other significant information. Your ability to connect information to other things will drive the information deeper into your memory. For example, if you are learning about accrued interest in a business class, you can connect the information you learn there to information you already know about your personal savings. Making the information more important and identifying its relationship to other things you know about—or connecting it to other needs you have—will help improve your retention.

You can also try heightening your psychic energy—and thus, your ability to retain information—by using one or more of the alertness enhancing meditations, movements, exercises, or other alertness tools you have learned in this book.

Distraction weakens your ability to store important information. Although all distractions are not bad and some may contain important information, distractions are generally (though not always) undesirable. They can result in confusion and scatteredness, and weak *sustained attention* and consumption of psychic and physical energy. Depending on the specific distraction—and especially if it is emotionally driven—it can attach you to other thoughts, feelings, and data, sending you further downstream, derailing your focus and sustained attention, and consuming the energy you need to encode a solid memory. Distractions can be external and internal—look in both directions, relax, and step back. Use one of your power words to refresh and channel your energy.

Once you've done this, ask yourself, *What's going on? Where are the interruptions coming from?* Consider, for example, if they are driven by some aspect of your environment or if they are internal. Perhaps they are driven from a lack of understanding regarding the information, or by something you are feeling physically or emotionally, such as a sense of urgency, apprehension, or stress. Consider if any of the distractions coming to your attention contain essential information. Refresh your mind, and decide what incoming information you need to activate and what to inhibit.

When a distraction is emotional, use your energy tools to regulate it and to deactivate its input. When your distraction is sparking from a lack of internal peace, identify the distraction as precisely as you can, then consider the difference between what you need and what you desire from the situation. Try using meditation (with your best calming sound or music) to help you connect with and feel into the peaceful energy of Universal values (honesty, compassion, acceptance, peace, and unconditional love) and full-being (tri-level) consciousness of body-mind-spirit. From there, you can condense and rechannel these energies, using them to "take the edge off" and help guide you toward acquiring what you need—and away from superficial desires.

Multitasking can thin down your attention to the point that your ability to stay focused and depot information in your memory becomes weak. Multitasking is sometimes okay and necessary. When it works, the tasks you are energetically involved in are often related—e.g., you are adding ingredients into a mixing bowl for apple-pie filling as you are also paying attention to your partner who is reading you the order and amount of ingredients. Because of the close relationship between such tasks, you can handle switching your attention from mixing ingredients to listening. However, if you are keeping an eye out for your exit on the interstate and are engaged in a conversation with your business partner on controversial specifics of a sales contract, it is easy to get distracted enough to not only miss your turnoff but also be unable to effectively recall the contract information later. This is the kind of multitasking you do not want to be doing when trying to ingrain material for later recall.

To help avoid harmful distractions, consider whether the activities you are simultaneously working on are related. As we have said, similar activities go well together. If they are not similar, though, try placing the related ones together and then prioritizing a list of things to do.

Achieving good memory storage can be compromised by attempting to process too much information. This sends your mind's attention network into overload. As we said earlier in this chapter, you can only focus on a certain amount of information before you overwhelm your capacity to store data. One way to avoid this is to consider what information is essential to accomplishing your immediate task, which allows you to focus on inputting that information and then use it to execute the task. After the task is complete, it is important to refresh your focus by emptying your mind and eliminating unnecessary information, which will prepare you so that you are ready to go again. Once you ingrain this energetic pattern, it keeps you from becoming scattered or confused, and puts you in a good mind-set when you want to commit information to memory.

As you work to improve your memory, it is important to note that information that has been intentionally inhibited or ignored will be more difficult to recall the next time around. The more you inhibit it, the harder the recall. So you may need to give yourself more attention and focus to make the necessary adjustments to the previously inhibited information that you now want to commit to memory. One strategy that can help is giving yourself a good retrieval cue to attach to the previously inhibited or ignored information. For instance, an individual I know uses color coding to remember books she has located in her bookcases: the red-book-cover section, yellow, black, and so on. This helps her find them more quickly. In your own life, you might find that organizing your grocery list with cues such as "breakfast," "snacks," and "dinner," will help you remember what you need from the store.

The anthem "use it or lose it" plays into memory loss. As we have said, repetition is a language your mind understands—it sends your mind the message that you want to remember a certain piece of information. So if you want to recall a series of chords on your guitar or piano, repetition is necessary at the learning point and also as time progresses. This helps create (encode) the memory and keep it from decaying. As such, repeating information you want to retain—especially at the encoding stage and then periodically thereafter—will drive the memory in deeper and quicken your ability to recall it.

Get Rid of Unwanted Memories

When an unpleasant memory invades your mind, it can disrupt a great mind-set, stress you out, and set you off in a spiral that will further lower your mood and cause even more stress. However, by combining various images from more positive memories, you can make fast and helpful changes in your brain's neurochemistry and treat yourself to an optimized mind-set. Then, by calling on these images whenever your troublesome memory bubbles up, you can train your brain to put an end to these nerve-wracking recollections.

To do this, you first need to identify the memory you want to replace and the circumstances, thoughts, and feelings that trigger that irritating memory. As you do this, it is important to also become sensitive to identifying when you are "almost" slipping into the memory. Be sure to consider all environmental and social factors, as well as what you were feeling both physically and mentally just before the unwanted memory arose.

Once you have identified both the unwanted memory and the circumstances that brought it to mind, it is time to make an entirely new memory to replace the troublesome one. To do this, use any of the positive-energy-building tools we have discussed so far, such as visualization, music, and massage, to intervene and shift your mind-set as the intruding memory comes on. If you want an especially invigorating experience, try combining sound, scent, and visualization to create a mind movie. This will trigger the release of dopamine into your bloodstream and create a feedback (reward) loop that will push your brain's reset button and get you back into a better mind-set whenever the painful memory invades. In time and with continued repetition, you can even stop it from coming to you altogether and keep it from recurring.

Whether or not you decide to make a mind movie, as you engage your positive energy technique, make it as sensory as possible. Feel into it deeply, and commit the experience to memory. Repeat this process whenever the old memory intrudes. With practice, you can deteriorate the troublesome and energy-draining memory and replace it with a new, positive, and energy-gaining one. Consistency is an important element when using this technique to eliminate the influence of negative memory. With enough repetition, you can train your mind to go there automatically—even if logistics mean that you cannot repeat the entire memory-replacing process.

Exercises and Practices

1. Use this meditation to boost your memory and place your mind in remembering mode: First, find a quiet place to relax. Put on a piece of calming music or use calming artwork you can incorporate into the meditation. Slow down your breathing and breathe abdominally. Let yourself feel relaxed all over. Think of a situation in your current life that brings you great joy. Keep a calm and joyful mind as the situation plays out in your head. Feel into the energy, and go with the flow of everything that presents itself. Visualize a few new ways to heighten the good vibes of the situation. See yourself flowing into these actions. Introduce a calming fragrance using a candle, flowers, or other physical item. Use this full meditation often, and your mind will easily associate this set of memories designed to sail you into tranquil pleasure. As an additional perk, when the situation you use in this meditation presents itself in real life, you will feel even deeper bliss.

2. Before trying to commit information to memory, use your power word(s); then play a power song in your mind. For me, Mozart's "Sonata for Two Pianos in D Major, K. 448" or Vivaldi's "Spring: Part One" (from *The Four Seasons*) work wonders. Remember: the more you love a piece, the better it will work.

12

Using Energy to Live Vividly

Consciousness, rather than being an epiphenomenon of matter, is actually the source of matter. It differentiates into space-time, energy, information, and matter. Even though this view is an ancient view, an ancient worldview, it is now finding some resonance amongst a few scientists.

—Deepak Chopra

Living a vibrant and brilliant life means consciously regulating and living into the energy that surrounds you; flowing within it, fully aware of being alive; unblocked at all tri-levels of consciousness; fueling and making creative choices as you leave one daily activity and enter the next. It is approaching life completely awakened to who you are, maintaining respect for others and being completely in the moment, happy and free.

The more you continue to practice and experiment with the energy skills offered in this book, the more effective you will become in accessing the energies of your full living being, your world, and the Universe—to help you creatively shape the life you want and the person you want to be as each daily journey begins and ends, and begins again.

Up to now, we have discussed various energies and a wide range of ways they can be used to address issues in your life: staying in flow; being alert, relaxed, and organized; strengthening your body and emotions; and so on. Now that you have learned these techniques, you can bring them to bear in a variety of combinations, creating countless possibilities for the life you want. You can change what you don't like, enhance what you do, and create what you have yet to attain.

Living this brilliant life, you will not get sucked in and drained by conflict as you encounter it. You will not fight fire with fire or beat your hands against the proverbial brick wall. You will instead use your energy resources to dissolve conflicts and exercise the power to remove yourself from gridlock when you experience it. You will replace the drains caused by conflict with energy gains, personal strength, happiness, and freedom. You will cultivate your mind to greater understanding, effectiveness, and future capability.

When you live this brilliant life, it shows in everything you do. Your life becomes a work of art—an energy unto itself that loops back for others to experience; affecting the shared mind of those with whom you live, the world around you, and the expanding consciousness of the Universe—all of which feeds back to you. This wonderful circle of energy is a celebration of your consciousness; who you are; who you want to be, can be, and will be. It is a celebration of your unique and creative life choices. It showers the Universe with you and the Universe through you.

When you live this way, you are the most animated and relaxed and connected; you are your authentic self. You use energy to naturally nourish yourself and offer nourishment to others. You have become the artist whose job it is to compose beauty in and through her own life—so much of which you can see is in your own hands and vision. You see and feel your presence, thoughts, words, feelings, touch, and movements—all of you—as vibrant energy interrelating with other vibrant energy. You make a difference—you know it because you feel it. You let the nurturing energy of other beings make a difference in you.

When you live this way, your excitement and joy for life is real and natural. It will come pouring out of you in every moment of living the masterpiece you are creating. You feel part of it all—yet fully you. Every brushstroke of your life gleams with energy.

As you live your vivid, brilliant life, don't forget to continue to practice what you have learned in the pages of this book. Foremost among these lessons is the cultivation of Self. As we have discussed, your Self (in the sense of "this is who you are at your deepest") is the hub of your full energy being. It is the headquarters of all your energy decisions and the source of your original, purest-energy default settings. Without being aware of Self, it is impossible for you to regulate the energy sources of your life so that you can reap the full benefit from them. Without this awareness and regulation, it is difficult—if not impossible—to know deep fulfillment, happiness, and connection with others in this lifetime, as well as with nature and the Universe.

Build on your introspection by making it a full being and regular practice, as we have been discussing throughout this book. From the perspective of holistic medicine and personal development, this practice is paramount. Softly advance yourself as you are ready. Live into all three levels of consciousness, and feel the informed power of their various energies shower through you.

Use and increase your empathy whenever possible. Don't just listen to others as they speak or interact with you; instead, feel them as they are present before you: acting and speaking and feeling.

Practice raising your sensitivities. Move your awareness of Self from the thoughts, feelings, and plans you have in your biological mind to your higher (nonlocal) mind. Get to know this higher-energy you better. Feel and see into this subtler, nonlocal mind (and body) and experience the space(s) it opens up to you. Some things will appear the same as at the physical level, but there will also be differences. Let yourself experience this new world. Have patience at this phase, and enjoy the vibrancy and brilliance of the experience.

Once you identify the dreams that nurture you—purposeful, exciting, Self-nurturing goals—build your scaffold of things to do to accomplish them. You will notice that the more you do this, the more you will shine from inside out and within all you experience.

Meditate regularly, and experience your original, true nature often. Feel into the energy of Universal Virtue and carry this energy into your daily life. As you increase your sensitivity to balancing the amount and quality of energy you are outputting with the energy you are inputting, you will hit your refresh button more often and more naturally. You will automatically recharge with the informed power you need whenever your overall energy drain is exceeding 20 percent. As a result, your body, mind, and spirit will feel lit with informed power.

Remember This

You are energy, your world is energy, and everything in your world is energy.

We began our journey through this book with the notion that, ultimately, everything, at its most fundamental level, is energy interacting with other energy. As you have seen, this connectivity has a powerful influence on us, and we can bring much goodness into our lives by learning how to use it. If you want to take control of and live your optimal life, you need to pay attention to how various daily energies are influencing you and how you can regulate them to increase the brilliance of all you do.

Our approach has been holistic, optimizing and utilizing energy at each level of the body, mind, and spirit. From the perspective of mind-body medicine, this holism makes our approach uniquely effective as a science, a medicine, and a life philosophy.

Enhancing and balancing the energies that affect your life will help you realize not just your physical, cognitive, and emotional potential but the potential of your full living being. It is my hope and wish that the concepts and tools offered in this book will move everyone toward this realization. The rest is up to you.

With practice you should begin to feel the positive effects of your endeavors very soon. And once you feel the difference, as a good friend of mine once said, "Who would ever want to go back?"

> Energy is the key to creativity. Energy is the key to life.
>
> —William Shatner

ACKNOWLEDGMENTS

I wish to thank my immediate family and extended family for their energies and guidance in helping bring this project to completion.

Special thanks are extended to my wife, Elaine, for the brilliance of her full, living being and for her love, friendship, creativity, and partnership along this journey; and to the beautiful energies that are our spirited and talented daughters, Isabella and Veronica, for all their goodness, magnificence, and peace.

Thanks to all my martial arts, tai chi, and chi kung associates, partners, and colleagues for their support, brotherhood, and sisterhood.

Thanks to Lon Normandin for his encouragement and support.

Special thanks to my agent, Linda Konner, for her great positivity and love of life, and for the energies of her insights and her ability to weave mutual visions into a collective, meaningful, and lovely reality.

ACKNOWLEDGMENTS

I want to extend special thanks to Dr. Jason Liu for his support, excellent teaching, friendship, and great energy, as well as to the rest of my teachers of philosophy, holism, and body-mind-spirit sciences and arts for helping guide me along the path for living vibrantly and happy.

Special thanks to my editor, Anna Noak, for her dazzlingly calm and analytical energy, and her outstanding editing and creativity—without which this book would not have been possible—and for her belief and support in placing its ideas into a public dialogue; to Sarah Heilman for all the ideas and contributions she made, and for her sharp organizational energies, guidance, and care in making sure the concepts of this book, which could get complex at times, came out as clearly as possible; and to all at Beyond Words Publishing, Atria, and Simon & Schuster for sharing this vision; and to the energy that touched me and manifested into the pages of this book.

It is with deep gratitude that I acknowledge my parents, Alfio and Josephine Cardillo, for their gifts of love and encouragement and life.

NOTES

Chapter 1: What Is Energy?

1. Lynne McTaggart, *The Field: The Quest for the Secret Force of the Universe* (New York: Harper Perennial, 2008), 33.

2. Lynne McTaggart, *The Intention Experiment: Using Your Thoughts to Change Your Life and the World* (New York: Atria Books, 2008), 12.

3. Deepak Chopra, *Ageless Body, Timeless Mind: The Quantum Alternative to Growing Old* (New York: Three Rivers Press, 1994), 14.

Chapter 2: Identifying How Energy Affects Your Whole Person

1. "Chakra Balancing: The Chopra Center at Omni La Costa Resort & Spa," The Chopra Center website, accessed February 12, 2015, http://www.chopra.com/our-services/medical-consultations/chakra-balancing.

2. Eric Chan, "Top-Down Processing and Episodic Memory," *Psychology in the News* (blog), Nicholas de Leeuw, November 25, 2007, http://intro2psych.wordpress.com/2007/11/25/top-down-processing-and-episodic-memory.

Chapter 4: Using Energy to Boost Alertness

1. Sonia Barrett, *Health: An Inside Job, an Outside Business* (Hollywood, CA: Timeline Publishing Inc, 2013), 115.

Chapter 5: Using Energy to Reverse Stress

1. Joseph Campbell and Bill Moyers, *The Power of Myth* (New York: Anchor Books, 1991), 183.

Chapter 6: Using Energy to Reverse Harmful Moods

1. D. C. Lay et al., "Behavioral and Physiological Effects of Freeze or Hot-Iron Branding on Crossbred Cattle," *Journal of Animal Science* 70, no. 2, (February 1992): 330–336. http://www.journalofanimalscience.org/content/70/2/330.full.pdf+html.

2. Rozanski, A., J. A Blumenthal, and J. Kaplan, "Impact of Psychological Factors on the Pathogenesis of Cardiovascular Disease and Implications for Therapy," *Circulation* 99, no. 16 (1999): 2192–2217.

3. Gayathri Vaidyanathan, "Stress Alone Can Lead to Bee Colony Collapse," *Discovery News*, October 7, 2013, http://news.discovery.com/earth/stress-causes-bee-colony-collapse-131007.htm.
4. Ian Sample, "Stress and Lack of Exercise Are Killing Elephants, Zoos Warned." *The Guardian*, December 11, 2008, http://www.theguardian.com/science/2008/dec/12/elephants-animal-welfare.
5. Jason G. Goldman, "Can You Die of a Broken Heart?" *BBC*, March 31, 2014, http://www.bbc.com/future/story/20140331-can-you-die-of-a-broken-heart.
6. Thomas J. Ryan and John T. Fallon, "Case 18-1986—A 44-Year-Old Woman with Substernal Pain and Pulmonary Edema after Severe Emotional Stress," *The New England Journal of Medicine* 314 (May 8, 1986): 1240–1247. http://www.nejm.org/doi/full/10.1056/NEJM198605083141908.
7. Moni Basu, "Why Suicide Rate Among Veterans May Be More Than 22 a Day," CNN, website, November 14, 2013, http://www.cnn.com/2013/09/21/us/22-veteran-suicides-a-day/.
8. David Rapaport, ed., *Organization and Pathology of Thought: Selected Sources* (New York: Columbia University Press, 1951), 58–79.

Chapter 7: Using Energy to Reverse Conflict

1. "1960s Tareyton Cigarette TV Commercial," YouTube, accessed January 16, 2015, https://www.youtube.com/watch?v=RB6C3o_-RdE.

Chapter 8: Using Energy to Reverse Detrimental Aggression

1. Mario F. Mendez, "The Neurobiology of Moral Behavior: Review and Neuropsychiatric Implications," *CNS Spectrums* 14, no. 11 (November 2009): 608–620, http://www.ncbi.nlm.nih.gov/pmc/articles/PMC3163302/.
2. John Gardner, "Moral Fiction," *The Hudson Review* XXIX, no. 4 (1977): 52–68.

Chapter 10: Using Energy to Enhance Physical Strength

1. R. E. Roberts et al., "Individual Differences in Expert Motor Coordination Associated with White Matter Microstructure in the Cerebellum," *Cerebral Cortex* 25, no. 2 (2012): 554–562, http://cercor.oxfordjournals.org/content/early/2012/08/08/cercor.bhs219.full#ref-45.

2. Tori Rodriguez, "Mental Imagery May Hasten Recovery after Surgery," *Scientific American* website, April 11, 2013, http://www.scientificamerican.com/article/mental-imagery-may-hasten-recovery-after-surgery/.

3. Ibid.

4. Vinoth K. Ranganathan et al., "From Mental Power to Muscle Power—Gaining Strength by Using the Mind." *Neuropsychologia* 42 (2004): 954, http://lecerveau.mcgill.ca/flash/capsules/articles_pdf/Gaining_strength.pdf.

5. Ibid, 954.

6. Colette Bouchez, "Want to Fight Fatigue? Here's What Kind of Exercise—and How Much—Is Best," WebMD, accessed August 07, 2009, http://www.webmd.com/fitness-exercise/features/exercise-for-energy-workouts-that-work.

7. Ibid.

Chapter 11: Using Energy to Improve Memory

1. Kevin James, "Phone Number Rhythm," YouTube, February 5, 2011, https://www.youtube.com/watch?v=iZfu-MtDsX0.

2. Christopher White, "The Smell of Commerce: How Companies Use Scents to Sell Their Products," *The Independent*, August 16, 2011, http://www.independent.co.uk/news/media/advertising/the-smell-of-commerce-how-companies-use-scents-to-sell-their-products-2338142.html#.

3. Joseph Cardillo, *Can I Have Your Attention? How to Think Fast, Find Your Focus, and Sharpen Your Concentration* (Franklin Lakes, NJ: Career Press, 2009), chapter 3.

GLOSSARY

active encouragement—a style of positive aggression that uses a mix of patience and calm to reduce conflict and inspire success

adrenaline—a stress hormone

alpha waves—brain waves that engender a feeling of calm alertness that is reflective and attentive

armamentarium—your available self-regulatory energy skills

beginner's mind—a concept from Zen Buddhism (also used in holistic medicine and arts) that says if you want to learn anything well, you must first attain the simple focus of an infant, whose mind is empty and fresh

behavioral tolerance—our ability to compensate for things that we expect to happen

beta waves—the brain activity of the waking state—the most alert state

biological mind—the mind associated with the body, also known as the local mind

body-mind-spirit system—your full, living being (see also *tri-level consciousness*)

GLOSSARY

brain waves—electrical currents in the brain

Bubbling Well—acupuncture point located at the center of the sole of each foot, about two-thirds of the way up from the heel to the base of the toes

chemical energy—energy that is stored in chemicals

chi—Chinese concept of life force energy, see *life force*

condensing energy—the act of summoning and compressing energy from your available resources

conditioned response—learned reflexive response to a conditioned stimulus

cortisol—a stress hormone

declarative memory—a type of memory that requires your conscious, intentional recall and involves conscious awareness and learning

delta waves—the brain activity that occurs with deep, dreamless sleep; the frequency associated with trances

detached mind-set—the calm, alert, and objective witnessing of internal and/or external life circumstances, data, and/or life choices

dissonance—a core element of music; refers to beats, sounds, harmonies, and rhythms that seem "off"—irregular or incomplete

dopamine—the body's feel-good hormone (associated with feelings of euphoria)

downward causation—the transfer of informed power from higher energy levels to lower energy levels (see also *tri-level consciousness*)

dysfunctional behavioral template—circuits in the brain that automatically fire our negative actions (habitual responses)

electrical energy—a current of electricity that is generated at the cellular level through chemical interactions

electrochemical energy—electrical and chemical energies or the interactivity and interconversion of electrical and chemical energy

emotional congruency—the act of matching pieces of similar emotional content

empty mind—a concept and technique that bypasses stress, attachments, and other negative feelings by emptying the mind of all negative emotions and thoughts

encoding—the process of taking information into the memory system for storage and retrieval

energy—see *informed power*

energy narrative—a method used to track energy levels and their relationship to daily/regular activity—how situations affect each other (past, present, and future)

energy templates—circuits in the brain that govern our actions (habitual responses)

energy trap—anything that depletes your energy

entraining—the synchronization of two or more rhythms, such as when the brain is presented with rhythmic stimulus from a musical piece and responds by synchronizing brain wave patterns to the rhythms of the piece

exercise addiction—a condition in which a person gets so involved in an exercise routine that there is no satiation point and the activity hits a level well beyond negative returns

fear-based memory—an emotional memory derived from a fearful experience; triggers fight-or-flight response

figure four—a martial arts joint lock that is launched against an opponent using either the arms or the legs positioned in what looks like the number four

flashbulb memory—memory associated with highly emotional, traumatic experiences

form—a term for martial arts techniques linked together and performed in a series

frequency—the number of waves passing through a given point, in a specific time frame (e.g., light, sound, or electrical)

functional distraction—a positive distraction

ground zero—energetic starting point

harmony—a core element of music; a parallel melody or cluster of notes played or sung to the original melody

heat energy—energy in the form of heat (also known as thermal energy)

higher mind—nonlocal consciousness (outside the biological body, also known as *middle mind*; see also *tri-level consciousness*)

highest mind—consciousness associated with your spirit (nondenominational; also known as *spiritual mind*; see also *tri-level consciousness*)

hubud—psychometer-movement energy drill designed to build energy

implicit memory—a type of memory that is virtually unconscious and emotionally based

informed power—another name for energy, which is composed of force directed by information

intercellular communication—communication between cells

intracellular environments—the workings inside a cell

ki—Japanese for chi, see *life force*

kinetic energy—energy contained by an object in motion

large muscle groups—the muscles of the legs, arms, hips, back, chest, and buttocks

life force—life giving energy flowing within and through all things; Chinese and Ayurvedic medicines, energy medicine, chiropractic, and other modern medicines address the use of subtle life force energy in their practices (also known as chi, ki, prana, and vital energy)

light energy—comprising particles called photons, this type of energy manifests both visible and invisible waves, and carries the full spectrum of color frequencies (red, orange, yellow, green, blue, indigo, and violet)

local mind—the consciousness associated with the biological body (also known as biological mind, lower mind, and physical mind; see also *higher mind* and *highest mind*)

lower dan tian—a major energy center in the body, located a few inches above the navel; your body's center of gravity (see also *upper dan tian*)

mechanical energy—energy that empowers your movement, potential or kinetic

melatonin—the hormone that makes you feel groggy

neurofeedback device—a neurotherapy device used to assist in the self-regulation and training of brain functions

neurons—nerve cells

nonlocal consciousness mind—see *higher mind*

parasympathetic nervous system—part of the autonomic nervous system, conserves and restores body energy (see also *sympathetic nervous system*)

perceptive filter—a way of seeing information carried in the memory; drawn upon to help you analyze and respond to events and other information

personal energy field—your whole being's energy

phantom stress—stress that results from getting worked up over nothing (also known as a phobia)

phonological loop—an aspect of your short-term memory that allows you to store auditory data such as verbal and musical information via repetition, e.g., repeating a phone number to yourself to help remember it

physical mind—see *local mind*

plasticity—the brain's ability to remold itself

positive aggression—compassionate firmness

posture—martial arts or yoga poses, positions

potential energy—stored energy that has the potential for work or reaction

power words—language that gives you the energy (*informed power*) you need for a specific situation

prana—Sanskrit for chi, see *life force*

procedural memory—essentially automated memory having to do with how you perform actions, such as riding a bike, eating with a fork, or even walking out of a room when a disagreement gets heated (also known as nondeclarative memory)

psychomotor movement—muscular activity associated with psychological activity (see also *hubud* and *Smashing Four Star*)

resonance—a core element of music; the duration or reverberation of a note

rhythm—a core element of music; a pattern or repeating beat

rumination—obsessive thinking about something such as a situation, person, idea

Self—who you are, what you are feeling on the inside

serotonin—a hormone sometimes called the happy hormone because of its contributions to sleep and good moods

Smashing Four Star—a psychomotor-movement drill designed to build energy

sound energy—energy related to the vibrations that produce a sound wave

spiritual mind—see *highest mind*

subtle energy—visible, intelligent energy found in the body and environment

sustained attention—the ability to stay focused on one thing

sustained exercise—exercise that lasts for thirty to sixty minutes and is undertaken at least three times a week

swarm energy—the combined flow of the strategic, coordinated energies (internal and external) that influence the personal energy field (see also *universal law*)

sympathetic nervous system—part of the autonomic nervous system, prepares you for quick-response action (see also *parasympathetic nervous system*)

synchrony—a core element of music; refers to the coordination of all elements of the piece

theta waves—brain waves that are associated with the deep, relaxed state of mind in which you feel somewhere between wakefulness and sleep; sometimes referred to as "dreamer's brain"

tri-level consciousness—consciousness within all three levels of the mind—local (lower/biological), higher (middle), highest (spiritual)—that allows you to mindfully explore your whole, unified life being of body-mind-spirit

Universal Law—the energetically cooperative nature of all things

untrained mind—a mind that is constantly allowed to attach to attractions (distractions)—what it likes versus what it needs (what is best)

upper dan tian—a major energy center located at the crown of the head (see also *lower dan tian*)

Virtue—a subtle energy that pervades and harmonizes the entire universe

visualization—a process using mental imagery and other sensory information to see yourself, someone else, a situation, and so forth within a specific experience, which may have already occurred, is presently occurring, or may occur sometime in the future

vital energy—see *life force*

white matter—the connective brain tissue that forms the communication network between various regions of the brain

working memory—short-term memory storage, short-term memory depot for information needed/used, for example, while carrying out a task

yang—cosmologically, the vital universal-male energy within all things (see also *yang* and *yin-yang principle*)

yin—cosmologically, the vital universal-female energy within all things (see also *yin* and *yin-yang principle*)

yin-yang principle—complementarity of the energy permeating all things, each depending on the other for balance